Neodymium-YAG Laser in Medicine
and Surgery

Neodymium-YAG Laser in Medicine and Surgery

Edited by:

Stephen N. Joffe
Professor of Surgery and Director of Experimental Gastrointestinal
and Endocrine Surgery, University of Cincinnati Medical Center
Cincinnati, Ohio

Associate Editors:

Myron C. Muckerheide
Associate Director, Laser Laboratory, St. Mary's Hospital
Milwaukee, Wisconsin

and

Leon Goldman
Professor Emeritus of Dermatology, Director, Laser Treatment Center
The Jewish Hospital, Cincinnati, Ohio

Elsevier
New York · Amsterdam · Oxford

From the Proceedings of the First International Nd-YAG Laser Society Conference, held on October 2–5, 1983, in Cincinnati, Ohio, U.S.A.

Published by:

Elsevier Science Publishing Co., Inc.
52 Vanderbilt Avenue, New York, New York 10017

Sole distributors outside the United States and Canada:

Elsevier Science Publishers B.V.
P.O. Box 211, 1000 AE Amsterdam, The Netherlands

Library of Congress Cataloging in Publication Data

Manufactured in the United States of America

CONTENTS

PREFACE

Lasers in medicine and surgery is a new and rapidly growing discipline. Recently the application of the Neodymium YAG laser has begun to assume an ever important role with a multidiscipline approach to its use.

The Nd:YAG laser was first introduced clinically for endoscopic photocoagulation of upper gastrointestinal bleeding. This proved in several studies to be highly successful. The Nd:YAG laser is now finding an ever increasing application in ophthalmology, urology, pulmonary medicine, neurosurgery, general surgery, gynecology, orthopedics and dermatology.

The topics covered are of current interest and have been chosen from an international team of active workers who are regarded as pioneers and experts in the field.

The results make fascinating reading and provide a blend of both laboratory work, clinical research and practical surgery. It is a major contribution to the current practice of laser surgery, illustrating well how fast the subject has been advancing.

We recommend this book to all physicians, surgeons, nurses, technicians and laser safety officers who work currently with or will shortly be related to laser surgery.

Stephen N. Joffe

CONTRIBUTORS

P.R. Abergel	University of California, Los Angeles Los Angeles, California
P.W. Ascher	Graz, Austria
G.W. Atkinson	Presbyterian University of Pennsylvania Medical Center Philadelphia, Pennsylvania
F. Aucomte	Department of Endoscopy Salvator Hospital Marseille, Cedex, France
P. Bailer	Frauenklinik vom Toren Kreuz Munchen, W. Germany
O. Beck	Neurochirurg. Klinik Klinikum Grobhadern der Universitat Munchen, W. Germany
F. Benech	Institute of Neurosurgery University of Turin Torino, Italy
J. Bourcereau	Department of Endoscopy Salvator Hospital Marseille, Cedex, France
J. Bourez	Centre Multidisciplinaire de Traitement par Laser C.H.U. Lille, France
R. Bowering	Urology Abteilung Stadt Krankenhaus Thalkirchnerstrabe Munchen, W. Germany
S.G. Bown	University College Hospital London, England
O. Braun-Falco	Department of Dermatology University of Munich Munich, Germany
J.T. Brown	University Neurosurgeons, Inc. Chicago, Illinois
J.M. Brunetaud	Centre Multidisciplinaire de Traitement per Laser C.H.U. Lille, France
R. Brunner	Department of Dermatology University of Munich Munich, Germany
L.P. Burke	University Neurosurgeons, Inc. Chicago, Illinois

x

Contributors (continued)

F. Carpentier
Laboratoire d'Anatomie et de Cytologie
    Pathologique C.
Lille, France

D.J. Castro
University of California, Los Angeles
Los Angeles, California

L.J. Cerullo
University Neurosurgeons, Inc.
Chicago, Illinois

J.R. Charlier
Centre de Technologie Biomedicale
INSERM S.C.N.04
Lille, France

J.F. Dumon
Department of Endoscopy
Salvator Hospital
Marseille, Cedex, France

B. Dupin
Department of Endoscopy
Salvator Hospital
Marseille, Cedex, France

C.E. Enderby
Molectron Medical
Sunnyvale, California

V.A. Fasano
Institute of Neurosurgery
University of Turin
Torino, Italy

D.E. Fleischer
The Cleveland Clinic Foundation
Cleveland, Ohio

F. Frank
MBB-Angewandte Technologie GmBH
Munchen, W. Germany

S. Fry
American Hospital Supply Corporation
Irvine, California

S.M. Gilbert
Molectron Medical
Sunnyvale, California

L. Goldman
Director, Laser Treatment Center
The Jewish Hospital
Cincinnati, Ohio

A. Gonzalez
Biomedical Engineering Program
University of Texas at Austin
Austin, Texas

A.A. Goossens
Molectron Medical
Sunnyvale, California

P.R. Goth
American Hospital Supply Corporation
Irvine, California

Contributors (continued)

D. Haina
Gesellschaft fur Strahlen- und
Umweltforschung m.b.H.
Munich, Germany

A. Hofstetter
Department of Urology
Municipal Hospital
Munich, W. Germany

F. Huber
Stradtkrankenhuas Traunstein
Akademisches Lehrkrankenhaus der
Ludwig Maximilians
Universitat Munchen, Germany

F. Jahjah
Department of Endoscopy
Salvator Hospital
Marseille, Cedex, France

K.K. Jain
Los Angeles, California

E. Keiditsch
Department of Pathology
Municipal Hospital
Munich, Germany

K. Kießhaber
Stadtkrankenhaus Traunstein
Akademisches Lehrkrankenhaus der
Ludwig-Maximilians
Universitat Munchen, Germany

P. Kießhaber
Stadtkrankenhaus Traunstein
Akademisches Lehrkrankenhaus der
Ludwig-Maximilians
Universitat Munchen, Germany

M. Landthaler
Department of Dermatology
University of Munich
Munich, Germany

M.A. Lesavoy
University of California, Los Angeles
Los Angeles, California

S. Bjorn Lundquist
Department of Urology
University Hospital
Lund, Sweden

C.J. Mackety
Director, Operating Room Services
Grant Hospital
Columbus, Ohio

I.A. MacLeod
Department of Surgery
Royal Infirmary
Glasgow, Scotland

B. Meric
Department of Endoscopy
Salvator Hospital
Marseille, Cedex, France

Contributors (continued)

J. Migne

Societe QUANTEL
Orsay, France

S. Mordon

Centre de Technologie Biomedicale
INSERM S.C. N°4
Lille, France

L. Mosquet

Centre Multidisciplinaire de Traitement
par Laser
C.H.U. Lille, France

M. Motamdei

Biomedical Engineering Program
University of Texas at Austin
Austin, Texas

G. Nath

Stadtkrankenhaus Traunstein
Akademisches Lehrkrankenhaus der
Ludwig Maximilians
Universitat Munchen, Germany

R.H. Osher

Cincinnati Eye Institute
Cincinnati, Ohio

J. Petronio

University Neurosurgeons, Inc.
Chicago, Illinois

R.M. Ponzio

Institute of Neurosurgery
University of Turin
Torino, Italy

R.A. Rovin

University Neurosrugeons, Inc.
Chicago, Illinois

E. Sacknoff

Harvard Medical School
Boston, Massachusetts

H.F. Schellhas

Department of Obstetrics and Gynecology
University of Cincinnati Medical Center
The Laser Laboratory
The Jewish Hospital
Cincinnati, Ohio

W.G. Solomon

Endo-Lase, Inc.
Washington, D.C.

C.P. Swain

Department of Gastroenterology
The Rayne Institute
London, England

M. Unger

Presbyterian University of Pennsylvania
Medical Center
Philadelphia, Pennsylvania

W. Waidelich

Institute for Medical Optics
University of Munich
Munich, Germany

Contributors (continued)

A.J. Welch   Biomedical Engineering Program
                                              University of Texas at Austin
                                              Austin, Texas

CHAPTER 1

EARLY DEVELOPMENTS OF THE YAG LASER

Leon Goldman, M.D.
Professor Emeritus of Dermatology
Director of Laser Treatment Center
Jewish Hospital, Cincinnati, Ohio

EARLY DEVELOPMENTS OF THE YAG LASER

Leon Goldman, M.D., Professor Emeritus of Dermatology, Director of Laser
Treatment Center, Jewish Hospital, Cincinnati, Ohio.

In 1961, there was a rush to develop new laser systems, Snitzer, of
American Optical Company, was the first to show the neodymium ion could lase
at 1060 nm. in both a glass and crystal host (1,2,3).

During the expansion period of the development of lasers, from 1962 to
1966, the concept of Movaki was developed of interest to the neodymium glass
laser by DeMaria, his associate at United Aircraft. This made for the development of Q-switched pulses, now important in the modern developments of the
clinical applications of the YAG laser. The pulses varied from 1 to 10 ns
(1,2,3).

The properties of the neodymium YAG at that time were power from 1 to
100 watts, continuous power, peak power from 1 to 10 megawatts, and beam
diversion of 0.5 to 10 milliradians. It was also during this time in this
period, that it was possible to get continuous frequency doubling, 530 nm.,
with the neodymium YAG laser using the crystal, barium sodium niobate. It
was also possible at this time to get some high pulses powers from fourth
harmonics with 265 nm. with 2 frequency doubling crystals and a Q-switched
neodymium laser. So from 1060 nm. with this laser it was possible to go into
the UV 265 nm. Q switching and mode locking (DeMaria) are of interest today
especially for laser ophthalmology.

It was found at that time, also, that the neodymium YAG laser, in the
near infrared, had a differential absorption of human tissues (4). This
proved of interest later on, especially in the laser treatment of tattoos.
In the early studies of the effect on the eye, the retinal absorption with
the neodymium laser is approximately 12% because of the pigmented epithelium.
When frequency doubled, neodymium YAG was used with a wavelength of 530 nm.,
the retinal absorption here was 74%. There was also a micro-irradiation with
Nd:YAG on tissue cultures.

The early clinical developments of neodymium YAG laser however began
with the eye. Zweng and Vassiliadis (4) on studies of the monkey eye,
found that with an exposure time of 0.6 milliseconds with energy of 4.7 milli-
joules that the retinal spot is in the monkey eye is 100 microns with the
retinal energy density of 59.8 j/cm^2. This produced a minimal reactive dose,
Zweng and Vassiliadis found out that with the neodymium that 30 nanoseconds
with an energy in monkey's eyes of 0.28 and in the man's eyes of 4.2 seconds,
the retinal spot was 95 microns with a retinal energy density of 3.95 joules.
This data should be of interest now with the popular use of Q-switched and
mode locked YAG lasers in ophthalmology.

It was also found in the early development of neodymium YAG lasers that
the protective glass needed for eye protection at that time was 2 mm. plates
of Schott glass type BG-18. This provided an optical density of 17.1 at
1060 nm. For eye protection at that time we developed a plastic eye shield
of acrylic plated in silver. The design was suggested after x-ray eye protection shield. Under 1% Pantocaine eye drops, this light weight shield was
used in the eye. Similar shields of light weight polished stainless steel
are used today for laser eye protection.

In addition to the eye covering, electric hazards were present. These
were high voltage 4,000 to 10,000 volts often used to store electric energy.

© 1983 by Elsevier Science Publishing Co., Inc.
Neodymium-YAG Laser in Medicine and Surgery, Joffe, Muckerheide, and Goldman, editors

In the early studies of Campbell (4) for eye disorders, he used intraocular laser fibers to produce specific localized effect in animal eyes. The green light of the Nd:YAG laser (530 nm.) frequency doubled was investigated for retinal and vascular effect. There were studies even at that time on diabetic retinopathy.

Our early studies some 15 years ago were with the treatment of metastatic melanoma and with tattoos. Specific absorption was found in metastatic melanoma masses and specific absorption was found in the colors of the various colors of the tattoos.

Safety programs were developed for the industrial and military application of the Nd:YAG laser. YAG lasers have been used extensively in metal working. Lasers also have been used for drilling holes in diamonds for metal dies. For safety, the observation of the procedures by the operator was on closed circuit TV screening, YAG lasers were also used for surveillance and for tracking planes, especially low-flying planes. At present, also there is extensive use of high output YAG laser systems in the military. There is considerable interest, not only in the communication techniques, but also in laser weaponry, not only for surveillance but also for alarms.

Our initial experiments on animal and human tissue were usually with 200 watts output.

With the special quartz fiber of Nath, our initial experiments with high output neodymium YAG systems were used for liver surgery as compared to the CO_2 for cancer, tattoos and even on port wine marks of man. In pigmented areas, there was greater absorption.

In our laboratory, the skin incisions with neodymium YAG were studies as regards the following factors:

1. The output

2. The optical quality of the target area

3. The speed of incision

4. The tension on tissue.

It is of interest that some of the modern videotapes that are being made to teach laser surgery use these same principles.

Comparative studies of CO_2 and YAG lasers were done for partial hepatectomy in animals. A special liver trauma device was developed to stimulate the trauma of seat belt injuires in auto accident. Then partial hepatectomy was done by Fidler. Capillary oozing was well controlled, especially by the CO_2 laser. Vessels larger than 2 mms. diameter required clamping. Nd:YAG lasers caused deeper necrosis in liver tissues than the CO_2 laser. Healing was excellent both anatomically and functionally.

Photovolatilization was done with basal epithelioma of the skin and with a series of tattoos.

In 1979, in vitro experiments were done with the YAG laser with fiberoptics transmission into thrombi capillary tubes. Thrombolysis developed. Microscopy was done of the impact area. At this time also, impacts were done on atheromatous plaques and also on crystals of cholesterol masses colored with various dyes for different laser systems and for fluorochromes. The fibers transmitting the low output YAG laser also were used to attempt to do

4

transillumination of tissue for deeper penetration in tissue than HeNe and HeCd. The object was to detect areas of different density deep in test materials and also in the breast of volunteer patients. Image converters were used to make records of these images. Also, special infrared photography, color and black and white, was used. The imagery was definitely inferior to the images of mammography and xerography. Detailed experiments were done in these transillumination studies by Greenberg and Tribbe.

So, this near infrared laser system was used in the early days of the development of lasers for the military for industry and even for medicine. Many of the early studies with their data can be applied to the current ever expanding applications of 1060 nm. and its variants such as 1320 nm. for deeper penetration into tissue.

REFERENCES

1. Snitzer, E., Glass lasers. Applied Optics, Vol. 5, No. 10. 1487-1489, October 1966.

2. Kiss, Z., Jr. and Pressley, R.S. Crystalline solid lasers. Applied Optics, Vol. 5:1474-1486, 1966.

3. Fountain, Wm. D., personal communications, 1980.

4. Goldman, L. and Rockwell, R.J., Jr. Lasers in Medicine. Gordon and Breach Publishers, Inc. Science, p. 15, 1971.

CHAPTER 2

ENDOSCOPIC APPLICATIONS OF Nd:YAG LASER
RADIATION IN THE GASTROINTESTINAL TRACT

Principal Author:

P. Kießhaber
Stadtkrankenhaus Traunstein
Academisches Lehrkrankenhaus der
  Ludwig-Maximilians
Universität München, Germany

ENDOSCOPIC APPLICATIONS OF NEODYMIUM-YAG LASER RADIATION IN THE
GASTROINTESTINAL TRACT

P. Kiefhaber, K. Kiefhaber, F. Huber and G. Nath
Stadtkrankenhaus Traunstein - Akademisches Lehrkrankenhaus der
Ludwig-Maximilians Universität München, Germany.

At present there are two groups of indications for endoscopic laser application in the gastrointestinal tract:
1. GASTROINTESTINAL HAEMORRHAGE, predominately acute bleeding
   lesions but also potential bleeding sources as in Osler-
   Rendu-Weber syndrome and angiodysplasias.
2. TUMOUR IRRADIATION as palliative treatment of obstructing
   carcinomas and curative treatment of neoplastic sessile
   benign polyps.

1. GASTROINTESTINAL HAEMORRHAGE

Acute gastrointestinal haemorrhage is a dreaded complication of gastrointestinal tract diseases, severe general diseases,
polytraumas as well as a complication of operative and pharmacologic therapy.
    The real danger in treating gastrointestinal bleeding
patients is demonstrated insufficiently by showing the total
mortality rate which is about 10% (6,15,16). But the mortality
rate of patients who need surgical therapy for their bleeding
control ranges up to 80% in varices bleeding and up to 65% in
ulcer bleeding, when rebleeding episodes are included (4,7,14,17).
Therefore a resolute approach in diagnosis and therapy is recommended. "Who acts promptly, helps twice" (2). That means to
avoid a greater loss of blood volume and the transformation of
the concomitant haemorrhagic shock into irreversible states.
The pathological findings of a haemorrhagic shock appear in the
first minutes after the start of blood loss in the shock sensitive organs such as in gastrointestinal tract, liver, lungs and
kidneys. These findings are manifested by changes in microcirculation (10). Disturbance of microcirculation in the liver, for
example, alters first the ability of the reticuloendothelial
system, ninety percent of which are located in the liver, to
phagocytize bacterias and to metabolize toxins resulting in
fever and sepsis (1). Therefore intensive care and medical therapy should be supported by an effective endoscopic method to
stop the bleeding immediately in conjunction with endoscopic
diagnosis. Using this logic the advantages are beside an immediate, direct control of success of the bleedings arrest, the
reduction of many factors which aggravate the concomitant shock
as duration of shock, the number of blood conserves, the con-
sumption coagulopathy and the number of emergency operations.
    Duration of haemorrhagic shock, which is of prognostic
value, can be minimized by the shortest possible time by occluding the bleeding source immediately after endoscopic diagnosis.
    Reduction of the number of necessary blood conserves is
desirable, not only because of costs and the danger of contamination with virus hepatitis, but by avoiding deposits of older
red blood cells and platelets in the nutritive capillaries of
the so called shock organs, leading to worsening of microcirculation (12).
    Consumption coagulopathy, in addition, can occur within
half an hour in severe bleeders, in recurrent bleeders or in
patients having a liver cirrhosis. Therefore the bleeding should

Neodymium-YAG Laser in Medicine and Surgery, Joffe, Muckerheide, and Goldman, editors

be stopped in time. Emergency operations in the acute bleeding state will be prevented, not at least in a high degree, if the endoscopic method is valid to stop massive bleeding sources also. On the other hand even short time operations worsen the conditions of the concomitant haemorrhagic shock, resulting in postoperative complications.
Laser irradiation offers the advantages of contactless application of energy, that means quick and exact aiming especially in moved targets, and of better controllable penetration depth of tissue necrosis in contrast to all other endoscopic methods as: injection or sclerosing measures and uni- or bipolar electrocoagulation with or without a simultaneous water jet.

Instrumentation and Technique

A Neodymium-YAG laser (λ=1.06 μm) of 100W output (Medilas MBB, Munich), a three channel endoscope (TGF-2D, Olympus, Tokyo) in which a special triconic quartz fiber for transmission of laser radiation (G.Nath, Lumatec, Munich) is installed, has been proven to work quickly, effectively and safely even under the dramatic conditions of massive bleeding (8).
An exchangeable quartz window protects the laser fiber at the endoscope tip to avoid contamination of blood and debris. By a third small endoscopic channel short pulses of a coaxial CO_2-gas or water jet can alternatively be delivered in order to remove blood layers overlaying the bleeding vessel tip during coagulation. The triconic quartz fiber has the benefit of a low divergence angle of the emitted laser beam of only 4.2°. This enables the endoscopist to maintain a working distance of some centimeters between the fiber tip and the bleeding source without a remarkable change of power density (Fig.1). The fixation of this fiber in the endoscope reduces the amount of handling and adjusting, allowing a faster and a more accurate shooting at moved targets.
A second,moveable gas assisted laser transmission fiber can be inserted in the most conventional endoscopes. The divergence angle of 10° of the emitted beam allows to vary the working distance only within a few millimeters (Fig.1). For keeping this fiber tip clean a continous periaxial CO_2-gas flow is necessary. This may lead to painful distensions of stomach and bowel, to embarrasment of respiration and to hypercapnia. Thinning the wall thickness by gas insufflation increases further the risk of perforation.

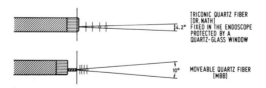

Fig. 1. The beam spreads of Nd-YAG laser radiation as being emitted from the fiber tips of the two different laser transmission systems: The triconic quartz fiber (Dr.G. Nath) and the moveable gas assisted fiber (MBB).

In contrast, only single, small volume CO_2-gas pulses are
necessary by using the three channel endoscope with the fixed
laser transmission system. Further, the insufflated gas volume
can be removed subsequently by the open suction channel in this
endoscope.

An augumented air insufflation pump has been installed in
order to compensate regurgitation of the insufflated air in
patients having a hiatal hernia or a bleeding source in the esophagus.

To overcome heat dissipation of absorbed energy in a spirting blood vessel and to create a sufficient deep thrombosis,
short pulses (o.5sec) of high power (80-90W) of a Nd-YAG laser
are more effective and more safe than long exposure and lower power
(<50W) or argon laser radiation (8). This experience has been
confirmed by R. Dwyer and others (3). By these short laser pulses of high power temperatures of 160-200°C will be induced in
the surface of a bleeding defect, leading to a glue like adhesive layer of coagulated tissue (Fig.2).

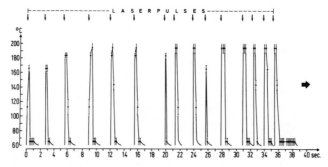

Fig. 2. Temperature peaks measured by an infrared converting
camera in the superficial layer of an experimental bleeding
ulcer irradiated by Nd-YAG laser pulses of 80W and 0.5sec.

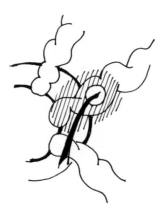

Fig. 3. A bleeding esophageal varix. At first the hatched area
should be irradiated to reduce the blood flow of the surrounding vessels. At a second step the bleeding point itself should
be coagulated.

9

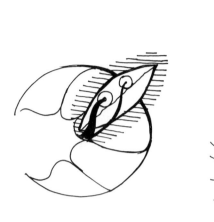 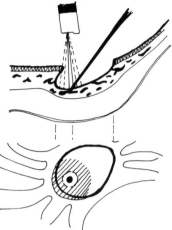

Fig. 4. A bleeding Mallory-   Fig. 5. An arterial bleeding
Weiss tear.   ulcer.
Fig. 4.and 5. At first the hatched area should be irradiated in
order to occlude the vessels of the submucosa. At a second step
the bleeding point itself should be coagulated.

The procedure of laser coagulation in spirting bleeding
sites of esophageal varices or arterial ulcer and Mallory-Weiss
tear bleeding should be aimed to reduce first the blood flow by
the CO_2-gas jet and by coagulating the blood supplying vessels
of the surrounding area. The second step should be the coagulation of the bleeding point itself as shown in Fig. 3,4 and 5.

In treating a bleeding patient, however, laser coagulation
of the bleeding source itself is an important, but only a link
in the chain of a suitable general treatment. Therefore before
and parallel to endoscopic procedures, substitution of the lost
blood volume is urgently necessary as well as restitution of
disturbed coagulation potential and avoidance of aspiration.

By using fresh frozen plasma and fresh warm blood for
volume substitution we had the benefit to restitute clotting
factors and unaltered platelets. This is very necessary in
patients, who have received analgesics or dextrans. These agents
result in platelet malfunction (11). This malfunction of platelets delays laser coagulation markedly and on the other hand
predisposes the patient for rebleeding in a high percentage.
Measurement of platelet aggregation by the Born-test or at minimum obtaining a history for the intake of those medicaments,
mentioned above, is recommended. Markedly reduced hemostatic
potential as in patients with liver insufficiency efforts substitution of prothrombin complex, factor XIII and antithrombin
III.

General anaesthesia with intubation to avoid aspiration
and to perform a better oxygen supply is not necessary in all
bleeding patients, but in shocked patients, in alcoholics and
in those who need a stomach lavage for visualization of the
bleeding site.

After laser coagulation reduction of acid secretion is re-

commended. Treatment by a combination of cimetidine and pirenzepin in order to avoid rebleeding was superior to a single medication of cimetidine or pirenzepin (13).

Patients

Of 1942 emergency endoscopies 1942 showed active bleeding
from different bleeding sources in the upper and lower gastrointestinal tract. This high percentage of active bleeders was due
to admissions of preendoscoped patients from over 30 hospitals,
who continued to bleed. These patients showed in 90% very critical conditions as a manifest shock (n=402, shock-index of Allgöwer   1), an excess of blood replacement (n=342,   1500ml within
12 hours) and a reduced hemoglobin index (n=282,   8g%).
The age of the patients exceeds 60 years in nearly 50%.
Severe underlying diseases as sepsis, coronary infarctions, carcinomas, polytraumas and severe operations represent further
high risk conditions. About 80% of all active bleeding patients
showed platelet aggregation disturbancy beside deficiencies of
clotting factors.

Results and Complications

Of 888 active bleeding episodes, 837 (94%),   according to
state Forrest I (5), in 692 unselected patients, were treated
successfully by Nd-YAG laser radiation. The reasons for failure
were: coagulopathies especially platelet aggregation disturban-
cies, technical difficulties and at times it was impossible to
direct the laser beam onto the bleeding site because of stenosis
or position.

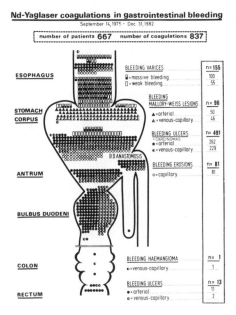

Fig. 6.   Topic distribution of bleeding sources successfully
laser coagulated. For each bleeding episode only one symbol is
listed.

The 837 successfully treated bleeding episodes occurred in
667 patients were (Fig.6):
  155 varices in esophagus and stomach
  96 Mallory-Weiss tears
  491 ulcers (included are ulcerated carcinomas)
  81 multiple ersosions and Osler haemangiomas and
  14 episodes in the colon and rectum.

Bleeding esophageal and stomach varices could be occluded
in 92%. Small numbers of thrombocytes and deficiencies of the
clotting factors aggravated the difficulties in stopping the
bleeding sources.
  In 30% of the patients we saw rebleeding from new defects.
Effectiveness of laser coagulation and rebleeding could be improved by transfusion of fresh warm blood. By this way the rebleeding rate could be reduced down to 17%. Two perforations
occurred.
  Naturally the portal hypertension should be reduced by
elective shunt operations or further bleeding should be avoided
by sclerosing measures after laser coagulation.
  The overall mortality rate in these unselected patients was
66%. The mortality rate in group Child A+B was 35.5%. Reduction
of mortality rate compared to results of emergency shunts which
are 50% (7), was not outstanding. But by a consequent consecutive treatment of sclerosing or shunt operations the result may
be improved.

Bleeding acute ulcers caused by stress, drugs, tubes or
other causes were difficult to handle because of severe underlying diseases as multiple traumas, operations or pharmacologic
complications. Difficulties in stopping the bleeding sources in
this group arose mostly from platelet aggregation disturbancy.
93% of bleeding acute ulcers were stopped.
  Rebleeding in all was 29%. The rebleeding rate has been reduced to 17% in patients who were treated consequently by fresh
warm blood and fresh frozen plasma. There were 9 perforations.
Reasons were: too high power densities in the spot size, technical failures or coagulations on the same defect in more than two
sessions. At the same time 13 perforations occurred in defects
without any laser treatment.
  After successful laser coagulation the treatment should be
conservative. An operation is indicated in deep growing and in
large ulcers showing a thick arterial visible vessel only.
  The total mortality rate in bleeding acute ulcers was 58%
when operation was the only available therapy in these severe
bleeders. This rate could be reduced to 30% by laser coagulation
(9). The mortality rate in the patient group which was treated
consequently by fresh frozen plasma and fresh warm blood was
23.1%. These numbers include all patients who died mostly
due to their intractable underlying diseases and not due to the
bleeding which could be controlled.

Bleeding chronic ulcers are more easily handled when compared to bleeding acute ulcers. Of acute bleeding chronic ulcers
95% were occluded. Five patients rebled. No perforations occurred.

  Therapy of choice after successful laser coagulation should
be elective surgery in all those patients having a chronic ulcer
disease. But operations can be done when the patient has re-
covered from the conditions of shock.

Mortality rate could be reduced from 25% in resection operations and 15% in vagotomy down to 2.9% by Nd-YAG laser coagulation (9).

POTENTIAL BLEEDING SOURCES

Potential bleeding sources as angiomas in Osler-Rendu-Weber syndrome which can be localized in the stomach and the duodenum as well as angiodysplasias, which predominately occur in the caecum lead to chronic anaemia. The surgical alternative treatment is total stomach resection or right colon resection. Because manifestation of both abnormalities occur in older patients the surgical risk is elevated.

Results

Eight patients having multiple Osler haemangiomas particularly in the stomach and duodenal bulb were treated by Nd-YAG laser irradiation in up to five sessions in each patient. Except in one patient no further operation was necessary.

Multiple angiodysplasias were treated in 22 patients by Nd-YAG laser irradiation using the CO_2-gas assisted moveable quartz fiber (MBB) with a reduced gas flow.
Except the first patient in whom the CO_2-gas flow of the fiber was to high, no perforation occurred. In all other patients no further operations were necessary.
No mortality was observed by laser irradiation of Osler haemangiomas and angiodysplasias.

2. TUMOUR IRRADIATION

Technique

There is a possibility of heat destruction of tumour tissue by Nd-YAG laser irradiation. Pulses of 80-90W laser output and exposure times of 0.5-1sec are used.

Method

Ablative Nd-YAG laser irradiation of stenosing carcinomas of the gastrointestinal tract represents a palliative treatment in order to relieve hollow viscus obstruction.
In the upper gastrointestinal tract carcinomas were treated in order to recanalisate physiological ways for better breathing, nutrition or bile flow.
Irradiation of early cancers in the esophagus and stomach is only indicated when the patient refuses operation or surgical intervention is impossible.
Acute obstructing colon or rectum carcinomas can be irradiated by using the flexible gas assisted laser fiber via a conventional coloscope, to relieve from ileitic or subileitic states. If recanalization can be achieved a preoperative peroral lavage is possible. This procedure allows to perform a primary tumour resection with immediate anastomosis opposed to a two or three stage operation requiring a temporary anus praeter naturalis.
Borderline lesions and wide spread sessil benign polyps as villous adenomas can be irradiated curatively after removing the mass of the polyp by a snare resection for gaining histo-

13

logical material. Sometimes more sessions are necessary to remove all the tumour tissue completely.

Results

In the upper gastrointestinal tract 14 patients were
treated palliatively: 1 cylindroma of the upper esophagus and
larynx, 5 esophageal carcinomas, 7 carcinomas of the stomach
and 1 carcinoma of the papilla of Vater.
One borderline lesion of an inoperable patient was treated
by laser irradiation with complete healing.

In the colon 13 patients with subileitic states due to
exophytic stenosing carcinomas could be irradiated. In 12
patients having exophytic polypoid carcinomas tumour reduction
could be achieved that a preoperative colon lavage was possible.
In one patient having an angled endophytic tumour stenosis
a perforation by laser irradiation occurred.

Fifteen patients with villous adenomas in the colon and rectum
were treated curatively. Three recidivations had more than two
sessions. Ultimately normal mucosa overhealed.

CONCLUSIONS

Endoscopic Nd-YAG laser irradiation for treatment of acute
gastrointestinal haemorrhage has been introduced since 1975. In
combination with restitution of haemostatic disorders a marked
reductions in rebleeding and mortality rate compared to surgical results has been shown. The success rate in stopping the
different bleeding sites, according to state Forrest I, was 94%.
Therefore performance of a controlled randomized study seemed to
be unethical, particularly because of many admissions of high
risk patients from over 30 hospitals in whom operations had been
refused.
Potential bleeding sites as multiple Osler haemangiomas
and angiodysplasias can be treated curatively by Nd-YAG laser
irradiation.
In stenosing carcinomas of the upper gastrointestinal tract
laser irradiation points out a new palliative procedure to relieve hollow viscus obstruction. Therefore insertion of tubes
in order to recanalize obstructed luminas were not necessary in
many cases.
Opening of acute obstructing colon carcinomas by Nd-YAG
laser irradiation enables the surgeon to perform a preoperative
peroral lavage. As a consequence treatment of primary tumour
resection with immediate anastomosis is possible instead of a
two or three stage operation with a temporary anus praeter
naturalis.
A curative Nd-YAG laser treatment in combination with snare
resection is possible in sessile and widespread polyps without
performance of operations.

REFERENCES

1. Allgöwer,M.: Schock. Therapeutische Umschau/Revue théra-
    peutique, <u>36</u>, 21 (1979).
2. Buchborn,E.: Handbuch der Inneren Medizin, Kapitel Schock
    und Kollaps (Springer, Heidelberg-Berlin 1960),p.962.
3. Dwyer,R. in: The Biomedical Laser, Goldman,L. (ed.),
    (Springer, New York 1981), p. 255.
4. Feifel,G., Heberer,G.: Die Problematik der akuten oberen
    Gastrointestinalblutung. Chirurg <u>48</u>, 204 (1977).
5. Forrest,J.A.H., Finlayson,N.D.C. and Shearman,D.J.C.: Endo-
    scopy in gastrointestinal bleeding. The Lancet, 394 (1974).
6. Jones,F.A.: Problems of alimentary tract bleeding. Rend.
    Rom Gastroen. <u>2</u>, 118 (1970).
7. Häring,R.: Chirurgische Notfallmaßnahmen bei der massiven
    Ösophagusvarizenblutung. Dtsch. med. Wochenschrift <u>102</u>, 289
    (1977).
8. Kiefhaber,P., Nath,G., Moritz,K.: Endoscopical control of
    massive gastrointestinal haemorrhage by irradiation with a
    high-power Neodymium-YAG laser. Progr. Surg. <u>15</u>, 140 (1977).
9. Kiefhaber,P.,Moritz,K., Schildberg,F.W., Feifel,G., Herfarth
    Chr.: Endoskopische Nd-YAG Laserkoagulation blutender akuter
    und chronischer Ulzera. Langenbecks Arch. Chir <u>347</u>, 567
    (1978; Kongreßbericht 1978).
10. Mittermayer,Chr., Ostendorf,P., Riedl,U.N.: Pathologisch-
    anatomische Untersuchungen bei der respiratorischen Insuf-
    fizienz durch Schock. Lichtmikroskopische und biochemische
    Analyse. Intensivmedizin <u>14</u>, 252 (1977).
11. Murr,H., Feifel.G., Schramm,W., Marx,R.:Zur Diagnostik und
    Frequenz der medikamentös bedingten oder mitbedingten, nicht
    durch Ösophagusvarizen oder Hiatushernien verursachten Ma-
    gen- und Duodenalblutungen.In: Blutungen des Gastrointesti-
    naltraktes, Marx,R. (Hrsg.).(Schattauer, Stuttgart, New York
    1975).
12. Neuhof,H., Lasch,H.G.: Hämostase und Mikrozirkulation, der
    Einfluß intravasaler Gerinnungsvorgänge auf den Schockver-
    lauf. In: Mikrozirkulation, Ahneleldt,F.W., Burri,C., Dick,
    W., Halmági,M. (Hrsg.), (Springer, Berlin-Heidelberg-New
    York 1974).
13. Londong,W., Hasford,J., Sander,R., Sommerlatte,Th., Überla,
    K., Weinzierl,M.: Kombination von Cimetidine und Pirenzepin
    zur Rezidivprophylaxe der akuten gastrointestinalen Blu-
    tung - eine multizentrische Studie. Z. Gastroenterologie <u>19</u>,
    514 (1981).
14. Orloff,M.J.: Emergency portocaval shunt. Ann. Surg. <u>166</u>,
    456 (1967).
15. Palmer,E.D.: Upper Gastrointestinal Haemorrhage. (Charles C.
    Thomas, Springfield Ill. (1970).
16. Schiller,K.F.R., Truelove,S.G., Williams,D.G.: Haematemesis
    and melaena, with special reference to factors influencing
    the outcome. Brit. Med. J. <u>2</u>, 7 (1970).
17. Schreiber,H.W., Kortmann,K.B., Schumpelick,V.: Indikationen
    zur operativen Therapie des peptischen Ulkus. In: Ergebnisse
    der Gastroenterologie 1977. Creutzfeldt,W., Classen,M,
    (Hrsg.), (Demeter, Gräfelfing bei München 1977).

CHAPTER 3

ENDOSCOPIC Nd:YAG LASER CONTROL OF GASTROINTESTINAL BLEEDING

C.P. Swain, M.D.
Department of Gastroenterology
The Rayne Institute
London, England

ENDOSCOPIC Nd YAG LASER CONTROL OF GASTROINTESTINAL BLEEDING

C P SWAIN
Department of Gastroenterology, The Rayne Institute, 5 University Street, London, WC1E 6JJ. Tel: 01-388 2411.

INTRODUCTION

Bleeding from the gastrointestinal tract is a common cause of emergency hospitalisation in gastroenterological practice. Epidemiological studies suggest that there are approximately 100 admissions for gastrointestinal bleeding per 100,000 population per year (1). In the United Kingdom, 30,000 patients are admitted each year with upper GI bleeding and 3,000 die as a consequence of this bleeding (2). Although there have been striking improvements in accurate diagnosis with the advent of emergency endoscopy as well as improvements in intensive medical and surgical therapy (3,4,5), the mortality from this condition does not appear to have improved and remains at approximately 10 percent in a very large recent American series (6) as well as in many other series reported over the last 40 years (2).

Rebleeding following hospital admission (7) is an important negative prognostic factor associated with a tenfold increase in the mortality; if this could be reduced by non-operative means, the high mortality from the complications of emergency surgery might be avoided. Nd YAG laser photocoagulation is one potential non-operative means of preventing recurrent or continued bleeding. The main theoretical advantages of Nd YAG laser therapy over rival endoscopic techniques such as diathermy are twofold; the bleeding is not disturbed mechanically during therapy and the amount of energy dissipated in the tissue surrounding the bleeding point is more easily predicted and controlled.

Short Historical Introduction

The principle of stimulated emission of radiation was predicted by Einstein in 1917 (8). During the 1950's, Townes at Columbia University and Basov and Prokhorov in the Lebeder Institute, who were working independently in the field of microwave physics, applied the theory of quantum mechanics to demonstrate that stimulated emission of radiation could be made available for practical use. They received the Nobel Prize for this work in 1964. The first practical laser emitting pulses of light was reported in "Nature" by Maiman working for the Howard Hughes Aircraft Corporation in 1960 and was a pulsed ruby laser (9). The Nd YAG laser was first described in 1964 (10). Yttrium Aluminium Garnet is widely used as a fake diamond substance and provides the necessary crystalline strength to withstand the considerable stresses of continuous wave laser light formation. The pink-coloured rare earth Neodymium, "doped" into the crystal lattice structure is the active lasing medium. When suitably excited electrons of Neodymium atoms fall to lower energy states, they emit photons of light of a specific wavelength which corresponds to the distance of the drop in energy state. The wavelength of light by Nd YAG is 1064 nm in the near infra-red portion of the electromagnetic spectrum. The same laser has an alternative harmonic emission at 1340 nm, but this is not widely used. The very high power of its emission in continuous wave or in pulses has made the Nd YAG one of the most successful practical and widely used lasers.

In 1973, Nath, Gorish and Kiefhaber in Munich first described the passage of Nd YAG laser radiation down an endoscopic waveguide (11). Two years later the first patients with gastrointestinal bleeding were treated

by this group with the Nd YAG laser. In 1979 Kiefhaber reported treating
in a personal series, 587 actively bleeding lesions in 459 patients
achieving 94% permanent haemostasis and also reported the results of a
laser coagulation enquiry compiled from replies from 31 groups using the
Nd YAG laser; 1776 actively bleeding lesions had been treated in 1533
patients achieving permanent haemostasis in 87% (12).

The Nature of the Continuous Wave Nd YAG Laser

The Nd YAG crystal is bombarded with light energy "pumped" from a
high power light source, usually a Xenon arc lamp. This input of energy
into the lasing material causes orbital electrons to jump to higher levels
of energy.   If a photon of light energy strikes an electron in this
high energy state, it will drop to a lower level emitting another photon.
In this way, the cascade of amplified stimulated emission is started.
The rare earth "Neodymium" 'doped' into the crystal lattice structure
gives the crystal its pink colour and it is the electrons of this atom
that are responsible for the laser emission.

Coherence

Laser light is particularly suitable for endoscopic use because of
its property of coherence - the tendency of atoms in a laser to radiate
their energy in a particular and defined direction, exhibiting the
property of coherence. Within the Nd YAG laser, the beam of radiation
reflects back and forth between two mirrors. The trapped beam has to be
carefully aligned since it must be perpendicular to the point of contact
with the mirror surfaces. This trapped beam then "stimulates" other
Neodymium atoms to emit photons radiating in the same direction which
means that new radiation is also aligned with the mirrors. By allowing
a small proportion of the light to pass through one mirror using a semi-
transparent mirror on the front of the laser, a coherent beam of laser
light becomes available for use. But since the large proportion of the
beam is reflected back and forth within the space between the two mirrors
(the optical cavity) the process may continue for as long as energy is
put into the system - this is the continuous wave type of laser, the
type used for photocoagulation. The tendency of virtually all the light
to emerge from a laser in a narrow beam makes for efficient focussing
onto an optical waveguide suitable for endoscopic use.

Wavelength

Lasers tend to emit light of a highly specific "colour" or wavelength.
The near infra-red wavelength of the Nd YAG laser light at 1064 nm is the
most important physical parameter controlling its absorption by tissue
and its consequent hological effect. Near infra-red light is scattered
more widely in tissue than light in the visible part of the spectrum so
the Nd YAG laser is the most deeply penetrating laser in medical use.
This specificity of wavelength of laser light relates to a fundamental
concept of quantum atomic theory, that excited electrons cannot increase
their orbital energies in a continuous fashion, but do so in quanta or
jumps. Emission of light consequent on a drop of energy state must be of
specific wavelength diffused by that quantum jump for the electrons can
only drop to a particular lower energy state which nature allows for it.

The combination of laser light with fibreoptic transmission

Endoscopists are familiar with the use of optical fibres for the
flexible transmission of an optical image. The ability of a glass

cylinder to trap and transport light is a result of the phenomenon of "critical internal reflection" (13). If a ray of light hits an interface between two dissimilar transparent materials, that light ray can be totally reflected if the angle of intercept is greater than or equal to the critical angle. Since light energy can be lost by being scattered by impurities which come in contact with the light at the boundary layer of the cylinder of glass or quartz, a cladding is normally used to surround the optical fibre to protect it from contact with such impurities and to provide consistent reflecting light. Without low loss characteristics, the passage of high power beams of laser light through optical fibre waveguides would cause an optical fibre to overheat and destroy itself. Indeed, when impurities of carbonised material or blood come in contact with the optical fibre at the tip of the laser, the temperature can rise until the fibre melts and is destroyed. Optical fibres of quartz or glass of 200-600 um are commonly used for laser endoscopy. Fibres of 1000 um are too stiff for endoscopic use. It is technically difficult to construct a Nd YAG laser with a minimal spot size of 200 um or less. The larger diameter fibres are generally preferred because they provide easy alignment of the spot with the fibre's entrance 'pupil' (14).

The endoscopic Nd YAG laser delivery system

The cladded optical fibre waveguide is passed through a loose protective outer plastic tube casing which allows passage of carbon dioxide coaxial to the fibre. The distal end of the fibre has to be maintained as a smooth optical working surface and is protected by a metal guard. The earliest waveguide to be used by Nath et al (11) was an ingenious but rather fragile triconic fibreoptic system designed at the Max Planck Institute which was incorporated within a specially designed endoscope, the waveguide being protected by a quartz window at the distal end of the endoscope. This fibre allowed a very narrow 4° angle of divergence of laser light as it emerged from the endoscope. Although there is some experimental evidence that this small degree of divergence may offer certain advantages in controlling bleeding since the smaller the angle of divergence, the less critical is the distance of the waveguide from the bleeding point, in practice this waveguide has been superceded by the use of much smaller quartz or glass single fibres of 200-600 microns which can be passed down the biopsy channels of standard endoscopes. The laser light emerges from these fibres at approximately 10°.

AIMING. The auxiliary laser

Because the Nd YAG laser is not visible to the human eye, another light source has to be used for aiming. For this purpose, a low power (approx 5mW) helium-neon laser is coupled into the beam path operating at 0.633 um which is in the visible (red) part of the spectrum. Possible disadvantages of this system are that the red light does not provide strong contrast with a red background, during the photocoagulation of bleeding, and the spot size of an auxiliary laser is not necessarily the same as that of the coagulating Nd YAG laser. However, in practice, it is reasonably effective for accurate targeting.

The technique of laser endoscopy in gastrointestinal bleeding

The patients are endoscoped as soon as possible after admission preferably on their way from casualty to the ward. The laser is left running during the procedure, having been tuned to give appropriate power and pulse duration before the patient is intubated. During the endoscopy, particular attention is given to identification and preparation of the bleeding site for treatment. Loose overlying clot should be removed by gentle endoscopic washing using a syringe full of water attached to the biopsy channel or to a washing catheter of "pipe" inserted through the biopsy channel and aimed at loose clot or debris in the ulcer base. We have not observed this technique to cause arterial haemorrhage. Clearing clot facilitates the recognition of the precise source of bleeding within an ulcer and is particularly helpful in deciding if active bleeding is present or not - often a difficult decision when there is oozing or intermittent bleeding. Overlying clot can absorb laser energy and prevent penetration to the bleeding vessel.

Once the bleeding point is identified, the laser waveguide is passed through the biopsy channel. The helium-neon beam is identified and is pointed at the target. Ideally, the probe is held a centimetre from the bleeding point but guessing distance at endoscopy is not easy. One technique which may help is to advance the fibre until it just or almost touches the lesion and then withdraw the fibre 10 mm through the biopsy channel holding the endoscope steady.

Most laser endoscopists profess to fire 6 or 8 pulses or laser energy to form a tight ring around the bleeding vessel. This is thought to increase the chances of thermally damaging the bleeding artery distally and proximally to the bleeding point, and may diminish the chances of causing or increasing arterial haemorrhage which occasionally may occur if the laser is fired directly at an unstable plug of clot or pseudo-aneurysm protruding from a bleeding point. There are no animal studies to support this particular treatment technique and in practice it is often hard to place each shot exactly, because the target moves. Movement can be controlled to some degree by giving buscopan and glucagon judiciously if peristalsis is a problem; inviting the patient to hold his breath while the laser is fired may assist if respiration is interfering with the aim.

Major upper gastrointestinal bleeding from ulcers is common in two sites, the posterior aspect of the high lesser curve and the postero-inferior aspect of the duodenal bulb. Both these sites can be difficult to treat and are usually approached at acute angles of between 45° and 0° using forward viewing endoscopes. On the high lesser curve, access is frequently improved by curving the endoscope with a J manoeuvre, and rotation of the endoscope with its eccentrically placed biopsy channel sometimes may give a different more useful angle of approach. Just occasionally, side viewing endoscopes will bring an otherwise inaccessible lesion into laser focus. Duodenal deformity is the commonest cause of inaccessibility. The use of an initial "sighter" spot on the edge of the ulcer may be helpful allowing a biological test of the lasers function. At effective coagulative powers, a single pulse should produce a ring of blanched mucosa but should not break the surface of the mucosa. Surface blood will be instantly charred. If the helium-neon aiming beam disappears or cannot be seen, it is usually wise to withdraw the fibre without firing it and cleaning any blood or adherent mucus from the tip. The laser tip can be destroyed by firing it when it is contaminated.

Laser Safety (15,16)

The main theoretical risk to patients is that of perforating a viscus. The reported incidence of approximately 1% with Nd YAG users is perhaps acceptably low in that these patients are hospitalised, closely observed and might well without laser therapy require surgery. The incidence of perforation may improve now that there is more information from animal studies on safe therapeutic parameters (patients with perforated ulcers will occasionally present with symptoms of upper gastrointestinal haemorrhage as well as signs of perforation).

Other complications include causing acute haemorrhage from a non-bleeding visible vessel (17) and possibly delayed haemorrhage (18). Discomfort from gaseous distension can occur. Low coaxial CO_2 flows are preferred except in the uncommon situation of spurting arterial haemorrhage, if there is any doubt that the gas escape mechanism is working, it is wise to withdraw the fibre and decompress the viscus. Metal tips are occasionally dropped inside patient's stomachs, but will emerge in the stool without sequelae.

The main risk to the endoscopist or to others in the room during endoscopy is of inadvertent eye damage. One endoscopist has already reported causing a scotoma on his retina using the Nd YAG laser. The Nd YAG laser used for photocoagulation of gastrointestinal bleeding is a 'Class 4' laser denoting a laser or laser system that can produce a hazard not only from direct or specular reflections, but also from a diffuse reflection. In addition, such lasers may produce fire hazards and skin hazards. Since light energy of the YAG laser is in the invisible part of the spectrum, the eye will not tend to blink when the laser light strikes the retina. A fair proportion of the light energy may be scattered in a backwards direction, i.e. back towards the endoscopist's eye. Many safety systems are currently used, either marketed by the firms making the lasers or devised by hospital laser safety officers; none are foolproof but effective protection can be relatively easily maintained with responsible usage and current experience suggests that laser usage is not likely to produce a generation of one-eyed endoscopists. The incorporation of filter for infra-red light within the endoscope will protect the endoscopist. If the laser system is used in a situation where direct or specular reflections are a potential hazard, staff and patients must wear eye protection.

Practical Problems associated with Nd YAG Laser Endoscopy

The problems that will be involved in installing a laser unit in a GI Unit will include finance. Laser systems currently cost between £30,000 to £60,000. They require a 3-phase electrical supply, some requiring high voltage. A high flow water cooling system may have to be plumbed in which may occasionally flood the endoscopy room floor. Because of the electric supply and water supply, lasers are not portable at present and patients have to be moved to the laser. Those patients most urgently in need of emergency treatment are likely to be those least safe to transport.

To maintain acceptable power outputs some laser systems require periodic maintenance, particularly to tune up the optical performance. The main technical problems of using lasers in conjunction with endoscopes relate to the fragility of current generation of waveguides. The commor causes of tip destruction include forgetting to turn the coaxial gas on, or the cylinder running out during use and unexpected contact of the gut wall with the laser tip when it is fired. This is usually associated with a characteristic smell of burning plastic coming up from the patient. Replacement fibres for some systems are expensive, costing from £200-£500; some have the advantage that the tip can be replaced by the user.

The Nd YAG laser is used with a coaxial CO_2 gas jet system. This serves to "back pressure" the blood spurting from an ulcer to clean and cool the tip and in the colon to prevent possible explosion. Kiefhaber et al have reported a marked reduction in the number of Nd YAG laser pulses required for treatment of bleeding lesions when coaxial CO_2 was added (19). Animal studies strongly support the hypothesis that coaxial

CO_2 enhances efficacy of haemostasis with the superficially penetrating Argon laser (20). Clinical studies with the Nd YAG laser do not strongly support the same hypothesis (21). The gas needs to be removed in some way to prevent overdistension. This may be achieved using a two-channel endoscope with one channel to pass the laser waveguide and the second to remove the gas. Alternatively, passage of a small bore nasogastric tube down by the side of a conventional smaller one channel endoscope may allow for greater manoeuverability. Not all laser systems can pass through the small 2.2 mm biopsy channel in 'paediatric' endoscopes, although now larger channel 'paediatric' (9 mm) diameter endoscopes are available. Some laser systems require that an endoscope be dedicated to laser use, to have an optical safety filter inserted into the eyepiece and a waveguide cut to its particular length.

Interaction of Laser Light with Biological Tissue

The most important interaction of laser radiation with tissue is the absorption of the light by the tissue with the consequent conversion of the light energy to heat the point or small area where the laser beam hits the tissue. The effect of heat on tissue varies with the temperature achieved. Between 37°C to 60°C simple heating occurs with a consequent speeding of temperature dependent enzyme reaction and altered water permeability characteristics. Between 60-70°C, denaturation of protein occurs with loss of cell membrane integrity and alterations in the form of structural proteins. At 100°, boiling of tissue water occurs causing cells to explode, and at higher temperatures carbonisation with charring is observed. The observed effects are those seen in heating a piece of steak with slight local swelling as membrane integrity is lost, the appearance of opalescence as proteins lose their tertiary structure, contraction mainly due to alterations of fibrous tissue proteins, the crackling or spitting as cells swell and explode (called the 'popcorn effect' in American literature), dehydration and further loss of volume as evaporation takes place as the temperature exceeds 100°C followed by vaporisation to steam, carbonisation and charring occur, leading to loss of mechanical strength at 400°C and the tissue may catch fire between 600-1000°C.

It remains uncertain which of these effects is responsible for the coagulation properties of heat. Vessel shrinkage is probably important in producing initial instantaneous haemostasis. It has been doubtfully suggested that local oedema disturbing the patency of the bleeding vessel may be of importance. Heat damage to vascular endothelium may activate the coagulation cascade and produce secondary intravascular thrombosis, but histology suggests that this may take hours to develop while the usual coagulative effect on experimental bleeding ulcers is instantaneous.

There is a limit to the size of external vessel that can be occluded by laser. Vessels greater than one mm in diameter are sealed with increasing difficulty, although small holes in large vessels such as the aorta or inferior vena cava can be reliably sealed without occluding the whole vessel. The matrix in which the vessel lies and in particular the amount of contractable fibrous tissue in proximity to the vessel probably also contribute to the effectiveness of haemostasis.

Animal Studies of Nd YAG Laser Photocoagulation

The clinical practice of Nd YAG laser photocoagulation is based on animal studies by a number of groups who have mostly used the standard (Seattle) model of gastrointestinal bleeding in canine mucosa, in which 1 cm diameter acute ulcers are induced using a suction biopsy capsule, the Quinton ulcer maker which cuts through an average of 5 bleeding vessels and bleed profusely in these heparinised dogs. The results of these animal studies are presented here. Silverstein in Seattle (20) initially assessed the Nd YAG laser using the early 4° divergent beam using the standard experimental gastric ulcer model. Their results are tabulated and discussed below:

Studies of Power and Efficacy

	15 w	30 w	55 w
Stopped bleeding / total ulcers n/n	6/12	12/12	12/12
Full thickness damage %		17%	75%	66%

The laser was not sufficiently effective at 15 watts but became effective at 30-55 watts. However, both these settings produced full thickness damage in two thirds to three-quarters of ulcers treated.

Studies varying Laser Pulse Duration

Using 55 w of power, the laser pulse duration was varied using 0.5 seconds with 5 seconds of delay between pulses to allow cooling; one second pulses without "obligate" cooling interval or continuous laser exposure to achieve haemostasis.

DURATION

	0.5 sec with 5 sec cooling interval	1.0 sec	Continuous
Stopped bleeding/total ulcers (n/n)	10/10	9/9	11/11
Full thickness damage %	50%	66%	55%

Studies of the Effect of Coaxial CO_2 on Depth of Damage

Using the Nd YAG laser at 55 watts, 1 second pulses with or without coaxial CO_2:

	With coaxial CO_2	Without coaxial CO_2
Stopped bleeding/total ulcers (n/n)	12/12	11/12
Full thickness damage %	66%	66%

Coaxial CO_2 in these experiments did not reduce the depth of injury (or significantly improve haemostasis efficacy).

Studies of the Relationship of Nd YAG Tissue Damage and Perforation

In clinical practice, the depth of histological damage is not important provided perforation is not produced. Dixon in Salt Lake City studied the effect of the 55 watt Nd YAG laser in standard experimental ulcers and produced interesting data on this topic. In 19 ulcers, a free perforation was produced with a mean of 9.6 ± 1.5 seconds (range 6.3 - 12.3 seconds); 13/22 had greater than 80% damage to the muscularis externa. There were 19 ulcers photocoagulated until bleeding stopped and then treated with 4-15 seconds of additional laser exposure. Fourteen of these 19 has greater than 80% injury to the muscularis propria. In their final and surprising study, a free gastric perforation was produced in 9 dogs using the Nd YAG laser. This iatrogenic hole was left open and the laparotomy incision was closed. All these dogs survived without clinical evidence of peritonitis. It will be seen from clinical studies that perforation with and without clinical peritonitis can occur in man. This study also confirmed the effectiveness of haemostasis of the 55 w laser in this model: 51 of 51 ulcers stopped bleeding with a mean time of photocoagulation of 3.56 ± 1.65 seconds; range 1-8.5 seconds.

Relationship of Power and Pulse Durations to Depth of Damage

Our group (22) reported studies of experimental canine ulcers designed to evaluate optimal pulse energy. Effective haemostasis required a pulse energy greater than 20 J. Thirty J was optimal except in the presence of spurting arterial haemorrhage which required 40 J. Optimal pulse duration fell between 300 and 500 msec. Shorter (50-100 msec) or larger (1 sec) durations were less effective. Using the Nd YAG laser with 75 w of power using 30 J pulses and a pulse duration of 400 msec to treat experimental acute bleeding ulcers it proved possible to terminate bleeding in a series of experimental ulcers staying within the safe limit for full thickness injury. Escourrou in France also studied efficacy and injury at a similar optimal power level (80 w Nd YAG) and compared this to monopolar electrocoagulation in standard experimental ulcers.

	Nd YAG	Monopolar Electrocoagulation
Stopped bleeding/total ulcers (n/n)	30/30	28/30
50% injury to muscularis propria n/n	5/60	24/60
Average total time	5.4 ± 2	28 ± 22

This group concluded that Nd YAG was as effective as monopolar electro-coagulation but that it stopped the bleeding more quickly and with a significantly lower incidence of deep injury to the muscularis externa. Johnston et al (21) found the Nd YAG laser photocoagulation highly effective in stopping experimental gastric ulcer bleeding both at laparotomy and endoscopy. Optimal settings in their endoscopic study were 70 w at 0.5 seconds. Full thickness histological damage occurred in over half the ulcers treated even at optimal settings controlling power output, spot size, pulse duration and coaxial CO_2. Although increased total energy, larger spot size and longer pulse duration appeared to relate to increased tissue injury with Nd YAG laser treatment; total energy was the most important single variable; 39/69 (57%) of ulcers treated with less than 250 J had full thickness damage, while 58/78 requiring more than 250 had full thickness damage (p < 0.05 Fischers exact test). Their studies suggested that the Nd YAG laser was as effective without coaxial gas as with it. Successful haemostasis with endoscopic application of the laser required almost twice as many pulses than treatment at laparotomy. Modification of the Nd YAG laser wavelength to 1.34 um did not reduce tissue injury.

Studies in the Rat Stomach (24)

An interesting study of the natural history of Nd YAG laser induced ulceration produced by 80 watts for 1 second at 1 cm distance, confirmed that the ulceration in this animal, as with dogs, extended to maximum at 4 days, the ulceration being approximately twice that of the initial area of ulceration. Treatment with inhibitors of gastric secretion, cimetidine or 15(5)-Me PGE_2 was not associated with an increased rate of healing at the ulcer base.

The Effect of the Nd YAG in Pig Stomach

Virtually all the experimental animal data on the efficacy and safety of photocoagulation in the GI tract has been carried out in dogs where the stomach is somewhat smaller and thinner than in man. Silus in Holland (25) produced some interesting data on the effect of Nd YAG laser in the porcine stomach on normal mucosa and experimental bleeding ulcers. Powers of 50-90 watts, pulse durations of 0.5, 1.0, 1.5 and 2.0 seconds to total exposure times of 5 seconds were studied. They concluded that 82 watts of power was most effective. Haemostatic efficacy correlated best with laser power. In their bleeding model, 12 x 1 second applications at 82 w of power was effective haemostatically and produced the least tissue injury. They made an interesting observation that the pig antrum was more resistant to Nd YAG damage than other areas of the stomach.

In summary, all groups found the Nd YAG laser rapidly effective in stopping bleeding in experimental animal bleeding ulcer models. Some groups reported a high incidence of full thickness damage while others appeared to be able to limit the damage by selecting certain parameters of power and pulse duration. Optimal settings reported by some groups range between 70-82 w and 0.3-1 second. Animals seem to tolerate full thickness damage and astonishingly even free perforation without apparent adverse clinical sequelae.

Controlled Clinical Studies

The apparently brilliant results reported mainly from Germany in the late 70's aroused unrealistic expectations that definitive controlled trial results would be easy to achieve. The high spontaneous remission rate (80% approx) in UGI haemorrhage and its varied clinical pattern, on the contrary demands especially careful trial design and choice of null hypothesis, the entering of very large numbers of patients and effective prospective stratification concentrating high risk groups. Careful reading of all controlled trial results available to date in my view gives less spectacular but reasonably convincing evidence of clinical benefit showing that the Nd YAG laser can at least stop bleeding and significantly diminish rebleeding, i.e. continued or recurrent bleeding in patients with bleeding peptic ulcers, providing that trials are properly designed and sufficient patients are entered. No perforations have been reported to date in controlled trials with Nd YAG laser which suggest that this may be an acceptably safe form of treatment. In a small, early Scandinavian controlled trial (26), 161 consecutive patients were randomised to laser or no endoscopic treatment. The results are tabulated below:

	Pts	Treatment Attempted	Bleeding Arrested	Rebled	Emerg Op	Died	Pts dying with oesophageal varices
LASER							
Active bleeding	23	15	14	7	5	6	2
Not bleeding	43	43	-	9	3	5	3
CONTROL							
Active bleeding	19			8	5	5	3
Not bleeding	50			8	4	2	2

This trial may be criticised in a number of regards. First, power levels used only a maximum of 50 watts - subsequent animal work has shown power levels below 50 watts to be barely haemostatic even in the easily controlled standard experimental canine ulcer model. In their high risk group with active bleeding, 8 patients randomised to receive laser treatment did not receive such treatment because of technical difficulties. A majority of their patients died of bleeding varices. This trial showed no benefit for the laser; its authors conclude "the material is too small to make any definite conclusions, and further studies are necessary in which laser treatment is compared with an aggressive surgical policy with early operation".

In a thoughtfully designed control trial reported from Belgium (27), 338 consecutive patients were admitted. 152 patients were included in the trial (129 ulcers). Presenting the results in the ulcer groups (rebleeding combines continued and recurrent bleeding).

	LASER				CONTROL			
	Total	Rebleed	Surg	Died	Total	Rebleed	Surg	Died
Group 1 (spurting)	23	14	14	7	NO CONTROLS			
Group 2 (non spurting active bleeding)	38	2	1	6	32	12	4	5
Group 3 (SRH, not bleeding)	14	3	2	2	22	7	5	3

The rebleeding rate in Group 2 was significantly ($p < 0.005$) reduced in the laser treated group. This trial may have been disadvantaged by their local ethical committee's refusal to allow randomisation of the highest risk (spurting) patients to no endoscopic therapy.

In a controlled trial from Scotland, 29 from a consecutive pool of 698 patients admitted with acute non-variceal upper GI haemorrhage, 184 patients were found to have gastric or duodenal ulceration as a cause for the bleeding. 16 patients were found to have a visible vessel either bleeding or not bleeding and were subsequently randomised to active laser treatment or to act as controls. The results are presented below:

	Total	Rebleed	Surgery	Died
LASER	8	2	1	0
CONTROL	8	8	8	0

The rebleeding rate and need for emergency surgery was significantly reduced in the laser treated group ($p < 0.01$). Note that numbers on which this level of significance was tested are small, despite the large number of initial patients. In our Nd YAG trial (30), still in progress, 309 consecutive patients were admitted with UGI haemorrhage. 151 had peptic ulcer at emergency endoscopy; 99 had stigma of recent haemorrhage (SRH). All 82 with SRH accessible to laser therapy were included in the trial. The results to date are presented below.

	Total	Rebleed	Surgery	Died
LASER	41	3	3	1
CONTROL	41	18	14	5

$p < 0.001$ $p < 0.01$ N.S.

They show a significant reduction in rebleeding rate and need for emergency surgery. No perforations were reported in any of these trials. Some groups who treat non-bleeding visible vessels have caused spurting arterial haemorrhage.

These early controlled trials have fuelled some heated and entertaining controversy (31) and have earned thus far only very cautiously a welcoming peer review in the medical press (32,33). The reasons for this controversy are these: the conduct of effective controlled trials in GI bleeding is a relatively new venture in gastroenterology. Very large numbers of patients are required to test even the simplest null hypothesis. Effective endoscopic prediction of recurrent haemorrhage, essential for prospective stratification of the high risk patient is in its infancy. Widely varying patterns of recognition of a "visible vessel" (34) which is regarded by most as carrying a high risk of further haemorrhage (35) and "stigma of recent haemorrhage" (36). Technical factors may account for differing results, some groups stressing clot removal and preparation with gentle washing of the bleeding point. Total energy and energy per shot varies widely. Following more recentwith the advent of a new generation of high power lasers, most Nd YAG users treat bleeding ulcers with higher powers and shorter durations than were used 3 years ago. Finally, a new level of endoscopic expertise is required which demands accurate recognition of appropriate targets for endoscopic therapy and the ability to clear clot from the ulcer base and deliver appropriate levels of energy accurately to a target which may be distorted and darkly illuminated because the intestine is lined with dark blood.

In summary, the results of the first laser photocoagulation controlled trials appear encouraging but further confirmatory reports are required. The impact of lasers on the problem of gastrointestinal bleeding remains to be assessed, but it has to be admitted that not all bleeding lesions treated are immune from further haemorrhage, particularly if a large vessel is exposed in an ulcer. Several important clinical questions require answering. What are the best power levels and exposure times for use in the chronic human ulcer; they could be higher since the white scarred ulcer base will reflect more light energy backwards. Is it better to attempt to obliterate the lumen of the bleeding vessel or simply seal a hole in it with a single, perfectly aimed shot? Is it worth repeating laser therapy if a patient bleeds again? Are lasers more effective, more cost effective or safer than electrocoagulation? Prospects for advance in the field of gastrointestinal bleeding depend crucially on the execution of controlled trials. It is important that the principles of the conduct of such trials are supported by ethical committees and that those involved in their design and practice should improve on these early examples so that the common goal of effective and reliable endoscopic control of gastrointestinal bleeding may evolve through controlled trials with a demonstrable reality.

REFERENCES

1. Morgan A G, McAdam W A F, Walmsley G L, Jessop A, Horrocks J C and de Dombal F T. Clinical findings, early endoscopy and multivariate analysis in patients bleeding from the upper gastrointestinal tract. Br. Med. J. 2, 237 (1977).

2. Allan R, Dykes P. A study of the factors influencing mortality rates from gastrointestinal haemorrhage. Quart. J. Med, New Series SLV, 533-50 (1976).

3. Schiller K F R, Truelove S C, Williams G D. Haematemesis and melaena with special reference to factors influencing the outcome. Br. Med. J. 2, 7-14 (1970).

4. Peterson W L, Barnett C C, Smith H J, Allen M H, Corbett D B. Routine early endoscopy in upper gastrointestinal tract bleeding: a randomised controlled trial. New. Eng. J. Med. 304, 925-9, (1981).

5. Conn H O. To scope or not to scope. New Eng. J. Med. 304, 967-9, (1981).

6. Silverstein F E, Gilbert D A, Tedesco F J et al. The National ASGE survey on upper gastrointestinal bleeding. Parts I-III Gastrointestinal Endoscopy, 27, 73-103 (1981).

7. Avery Jones F. Haematemesis and melaena with special reference to causation and to the factors influencing the mortality from bleeding peptic ulcers. Gastroenterology 30, 166-9 (1956).

8. Einstein A. Zur quantentheorie der Strahlung. Phys. Z. 18, 121 (1917).

9. Maiman T H. Stimulated optical radiation in ruby. Nature 187, 493-4 (1960).

10. Gensic J E, Marcos H M and can Uitert L G. Laser oscillations in Nd-Doped Yttrium Aluminium, Yttrium gallium and Gadolinium garnet. Applied Physics Letters 4, 182-4 (1964).

11. Nath G, Gorish W, Kiefhaber P. First laserendoscopy via a fibreoptic transmission system. Endoscopy 5, 208-13 (1973).

12. Kiefhaber P, Moritz K, Heldwein W, Lehnert P and Weidinger P. Endoscopische Blutstillung Glutender Osophagus und Magenvarizen mit einem Hochleistungs Neodym YAG Laser. In: Operative Endoskopie (Demling L and Rosch W ed.) Acrm, Berlin (1979).

13. Hirschowitz B I, Curtess L E, Peters C W and Pollard H M. Demonstration of a new gastroscope, the "Fibrescope". Gastroenterobgy (1958).

14. Auth D C. Laser photocoagulation principles in "Endoscopic control of gastrointestinal haemorrhage" ed. J P Papp 1981. CRC Press, Florida, p 73-86.

15. Mallow A, Chabot L. Laser Safety Handbook 1978. Van Nostrand Reinhold Company, New York.

16. Laser Safety Guide of the Laser Institute of America. 5th edition 1982. Laser Institute of America, 515 Monroe Street, Toledo OH 43623.

17. Swain C P, Bown S G, Storey D W et al. Controlled trial of Argon laser photocoagulation in bleeding peptic ulcers. Lancet 11, 1313-6 (1981).

18. Johnston J H. Complications following endoscopic laser therapy. Gastrointestinal Endoscopy 28, 2, 135, (1982).

19. Kiefhaber P, Nath G, Moritz K. Endoscopic control of acute gastrointestinal haemorrhage by irradiation with high power Neodymium-YAG laser. Presented at the International Medical Laser Symposium, Detroit, Michigan, March 197-.

20. Silverstein F E, Protell R L, Gilbert D A, Gularsih C, Auth D C, Dennis M B and Rubin C E. Argon vs. Neodymium YAG laser photocoagulation of experimental canine gastric ulcers. Gastroenterology 77, 647 (1979).

21. Johnston J H, Jensen D M, Mautner W and Elashoff J. YAG laser treatment of experimental bleeding canine gastric ulcers. Gastroenterology 79, 1256-61 (1980).
22. Dixon J A, Berenson M M, McClosky D W. Neodymium YAG laser treatment of experimental canine gastric bleeding. Gastroenterology 77, 647-51, (1979).
23. Bown S G, Salmon P R, Storey D W, Calder B A, Ke-ly D F, Adams N, Pearson H, Weaver B M Q. Nd YAG laser photocoagulation in the dog stomach. Gut 21, 818-25 (1980).
24. MacLeod I A. Lee F D, Lewi H J E, Joffe S N. The effect of cimetidine and 15(S) 15-methyl prostaglandin E2 on the healing of laser-induced gastric mucosal damage. Gastrointest. Endosc. 28, no. 3, 166, (1982).
25. Sluis R F vd, Holland R and Yap S H. Experience with Neodymium YAG laser photocoagulation in experimental gastric ulcers in pig. In: Abstracts of the IV European Congress of Gastrointestinal Endoscopy, George Thieme Verlag, Stuttgart, Germany, 115 (1980).
26. Ihre T, Johansson C, Seligson V, Torregren S. Endoscopic YAG laser treatment in massive upper gastrointestinal bleeding. Report of a controlled randomised study. Scand. J. Gastroenterol. 16, 633-40, (1981).
27. Rutgeerts P, Vantrappen G, Broeckhaert L, Janssens H. Coremans G, Geboes K and Schurmans P. Controlled trial of Nd YAG laser treatment of upper digestive haemorrhage. Gastroenterology 83, 410-6 (1982)
29. MacLeod I A, Mills P R, Mackenzie J F, Joffe S N, Russell R I, Carter D C. Neodymium Yttrium aluminium garnet laser photocoagulation for major haemorrhage from peptic ulcers and single vessels: a single blind controlled study. Br. Med. J. 286, 345-8 (1983).
30. Swain C P, Bown S G, Salmon P R, Kirkham H S and Northfield T C. Controlled trial of Nd YAG laser photocoagulation in bleeding peptic ulcers. Gastroenterology 84, 1327(A) (1983).
31. Bateson M C, Henry D A, Langman M J S, Cotton P B, Vallon A G, Piper D W, Northfield T C. Letters to the Lancet 1c, 99, 172, 230, 231, 401, 508 (1982).
32. Peterson W L. Laser therapy for bleeding peptic ulcer. A burning issue? Gastroenterology 83, 584-88 (1982).
33. Anon Editorial. Laser coagulation in bleeding peptic ulcers. Passing gimmick or life-saving advance? Lancet 2, 804-5 (1982).
34. Griffiths W J, Neumann D A, Welsh J D. The visible vessel as an indicator of uncontrolled or recurrent gastrointestinal haemorrhage. N. Eng. J. Med. 300, -411-3, (1979).
35. Storey D W, Bown S G, Swain C P et al. Endoscopic prediction of recurrent bleeding in peptic ulcers. New. Eng. J. Med. 305, 915-6, (1981).
36. Foster D N, Miloszewski K J A, Losowsky M S. Stigmata of recent haemorrhage in diagnosis and prognosis of upper gastrointestinal bleeding. Br. Med. J. 1, 1173-7 (1978).

CHAPTER 4

Nd:YAG LASER PHOTOCOAGULATION FOR PEPTIC ULCER HEMORRHAGE

Ian A. MacLeod, M.D.
Department Surgery
Royal Infirmary
Glasgow, Scotland

Nd:YAG LASER PHOTOCOAGULATION FOR PEPTIC ULCER HEMORRHAGE

Ian A. MacLeod, M.D.
Department of Surgery, Royal Infirmary, Glasgow G4 OSF, Scotland.

INTRODUCTION

At present, emergency surgery is the accepted method of arresting continuous or further hemorrhage from peptic ulceration. However, many of the patients undergoing operation for this problem are elderly, have coexistent cardiorespiratory disease, and consequently there is an appreciable mortality (1-3). Dronfield analyzed the causes of death in a series of patients bleeding from the upper gastrointestinal tract and found that postoperative complications were the commonest causes of potentially avoidable deaths (4). If continuous or further hemorrhage could be treated or prevented by non-operative techniques, then hopefully, the mortality from peptic ulcer hemorrhage might be reduced.

With the advent of fibre optic endoscopy, therapeutic endoscopy became feasible because the site and cause of bleeding can be identified in a high proportion of patients (5), the procedure has a low complication rate (6) and in most cases, the endoscope affords direct access to the source of bleeding.

Neodymium YAG laser photocoagulation was first used to treat a patient by Kiefhaber in 1975 (7) and in the enusing eight years much experimental and clinical information has accrued and this chapter reviews the evidence for the safety and efficacy of this particular technique of therapeutic endoscopy.

THEORY AND EQUIPMENT

The mechanism of action of Nd:YAG photocoagulation depends on the fact that light energy when absorbed in tissue is converted instantly to thermal energy which is realized by a rise in tissue temperature (8). When the temperature rises above $60^{\circ}C$, coagulation of protein occurs. The distribution of coagulative necrosis in tissue is dependent primarily on the intrinsic optic properties of the radiation and the tissue it is incident upon (9). Because tissue such as the stomach wall is not a homogeneous medium, Beers Law does not apply and the radiation undergoes a redistributive internal scattering which produces an in depth volume heating (10). Nd:YAG radiation ($\lambda = 1.06$ μm) penetrates more deeply in red pigment than the radiation of the argon ion laser and is not well absorbed until a depth of 300 μm has been reached. Its radiation penetrates five times deeper in gastric tissue than that of the argon laser (7). It is thought that hemostasis is achieved by a coagulation of blood and a shrinkage of collagen which is an important constituent of a blood vessel and the surrounding fibrous tissue in an ulcer floor. In addition, there is a reactive edema to the surrounding tissue.

Nd:YAG photocoagulation is technically feasible because its radiation can be transmitted efficiently through a fibre optic which is small enough to be encased in a cannula that can be passed down the biopsy channel of an endoscope. Because the Nd:YAG radiation does not have such a high spatial coherence as the argon ion laser, the minimum fibre optic diameter that can be used is 200 μm. Unless a triconal fibre is used, coaxial carbon dioxide must be used to keep the fibre tip clean. The gas is also used to clean blood from the source of bleeding and if necessary, divert a stream of blood from the vessel. When coaxial carbon dioxide is used, a venting system must be used to prevent over distention of the stomach.

© 1983 by Elsevier Science Publishing Co., Inc.
Neodymium-YAG Laser in Medicine and Surgery, Joffe, Muckerheide, and Goldman, editors

Because the radiation of the Nd:YAG laser is invisible, visible target marker beams are used and the systems in operation are a helium neon laser (Messerschmidt and Fibrelase 100) or Xenon lamp (Molectron).

SAFETY

For any technique of therapeutic endoscopy to be clinically acceptable, it must not only be effective in arresting hemorrhage but also cause minimal side effects to the patient or operation. The radiation of the neodymium YAG laser has a relatively deep penetration into the stomach wall and thus there is the risk of visceral perforation and its attendent complications to a patient. Several studies have been done with Nd:YAG photocoagulation to assess the depth of coagulation necrosis in the stomach wall of an animal by using the quinton ulcer bleeding model and full thickness muscle necrosis was found to be common (11-14). In particular, Silverstein found that full thickness muscle necrosis of the gastric wall occurred irrespective of the laser power used, the duration of exposure, or the presence or absence of coaxial carbon dioxide, but there was no evidence of visceral perforation (11). The occurrence of full muscle thickness necrosis does not itself equate with visceral perforation, especially since the serosa may have an increased resistance to laser radiation (12). The experience obtained from the quinton ulcer model has to be interpreted with caution particularly when considering the potential risk to a patient who has bled from a peptic ulcer and might benefit from therapeutic endoscopy. In the clinical situation, a perforation could conceivably occur from irradiation of the intact stomach wall or the ulcer floor itself. In relation to the former situation, Kiefhaber found that perforation of an intact dog stomach occurred when the quantity of radiation used was seven times that required to produce coagulation of a bleeding point (7). With respect to bleeding peptic ulcers, the quinton ulcer has none of the features of inflammation or repair seen in a peptic ulcer. Stewart found that 28% of peptic lers are adherent to the pancreas or liver and that 42% of gastric and duodenal ulcers had adhesions. Patients who have bled from peptic ulcers and might benefit from laser photocoagulation have almost certainly bled from a single sizeable vessel in the ulcer floor (16), and in reality, the laser radiation is directed at the vessel itself and not the ulcer floor. The more recent experimental ulcer model with a single bleeding artery described by Dennis et al lends support to the last comment particularly when it was found that none of the sixteen ulcers photocoagulated had full thickness muscle necrosis (17).

The final evidence supporting the contention that the risk of perforation with Nd:YAG photocoagulation is low comes from the clinical experience available. By 1979, Kiefhaber had treated 627 patients with this laser and had reported six perforations (1%). Analysis of his data shows that in four gas insufflation reopened scaled perforations (0.6%) and in only two cases could the laser radiation be implicated (0.3%). However, in both cases, laser photocoagulation was used twice on the same site on successive days (18). Thus, when correct energy levels are used (for example pulses of 40 joules) the risk of visceral perforation to a patient with this laser is low.

It is worthy of note that the incidence of visceral perforation from diagnostic endoscopy of patients who had bled from gastric and duodenal ulcers in the National ASGI Surgey on upper gastrointestinal bleeding reported in 1981 was 0.5% (6). Because of the appreciable reflected and back scattering of Nd:YAG radiation from the stomach wall and possible transmission up the optics of the endoscope, there is the risk of damage to the operator's eye (19), however, this risk if obviated by the placement of a filter in the endoscope eye piece or by the use of appropriate safety goggles. A laser photocoagulation is performed in a closed situation, the risk to assistant personnel within the laser room is minimal.

EFFICACY

Experimental

Most of the experimental work done to assess the efficacy of Nd:YAG photocoagulation has utilized the quinton ulcer model and impressive results have been achieved (11-14). However, this model has several deficiencies in that the ulcer maker transects several small vessels in the submucosa which tend to retract under the ulcer rim. The rate of bleeding is low and variable and many ulcers stop bleeding spontaneously and therefore the animals are heparinized. The ulcer has none of the histological features of inflammation or repair seen in acute or chronic peptic ulcers in a patient. Thus, great caution must be exercised in extrapolating the experimental results to the clinical situation. Patients who have bled from peptic ulcers and are at high risk of further hemorrhage may not be bleeding actively at the time of endoscopy and tend to have a single sizeable vessel in the ulcer floor which has not been transected.

Other more realistic models have been described but none of them meet in total the clinical situation (17,20).

Clinical Experience

The Nd:YAG laser has been used to treat a large number of patients with encouraging results (18). Unfortunately, because of the natural tendency for bleeding peptic ulcers to stop bleeding spontaneously, it is necessary to perform a controlled trial to assess the efficacy of any endoscopic therapeutic technique.

Controlled Trials

To date, the results from three controlled trials of Nd:YAG photocoagulation have been published in full. Because the entry criteria used in each trial are different, their results cannot be combined.

The trial conducted in Stockholm by Ihre et al failed to show any benefit from Nd:YAG laser photocoagulation. However, the various causes of bleeding were not separated into different groups and no reference was made to the presence or absence of vessels and thus the efficacy of the Nd:YAG laser for bleeding peptic ulcers cannot be determined from this trial (21).

The study of Rutgeerts et al from Leaven in Belgium divided the patients bleeding from peptic ulcers into three different groups. The first comprised patients who had active arterial bleeding at the time of endoscopy. All of them received laser photocoagulation which was effective in achieving hemostasis in 20 (87%). However, 11 of them rebled and thus haemostasis was permanent in only nine (45%). The second group comprised 67 patients who had active but non-pulsatile bleeding at the time of endoscopy, and they were randomized to receive laser, 38, or Sham, 32, therapy. Laser photocoagulation produced initial hemostasis in all patients compared with only 25 (78%) of the control group (p < 0.01). Overall, only two (5%) of the laser treated group rebled compared with 12 (38%) of the controls (p<0.005). There was no difference in the requirement for emergency surgery or the resultant mortality. The third group consisted of patients who had bled from peptic ulcers and were not actively bleeding at the time of endoscopy but had either a red clot or a vessel in the ulcer floor. There was no difference in the outcome between the two treatment groups but unfortunately, the outcome of those with vessels was not determined and no description of a vessel was given (22).

The single blind controlled trial of Nd:YAG photocoagulation performed in Glasgow, Scotland, included clinical features in the study entry criteria, to select patients who were at high risk from further hemorrhage. One hundred and eighty-four patients who had bled from peptic ulcers and single vessels were considered, but 130 were ineligible and all of them received conservative management. Fifty-four were eligible and 45 entered the study. Twenty-five had ulcers with spots in the base and irrespective of therapy, all received conservative management. Twenty patients had bled from arteries and all eight who were allocated to the control group rebled and underwent emergency surgery and two died. Although 12 patients bleeding from arteries were allocated to laser therapy, four did not receive it and all of them rebled and had emergency surgery with one death. Of the eight who received laser therapy, two rebled and one required emergency surgery. Thus, of those who received laser therapy the occurrence of further hemorrhage and the need for emergency surgery was reduced (p = 0.01 and p = 0.001 respectively). Overall, the occurrence of further hemorrhage in the laser treated group as a whole was reduced (p<0.05) as was the need for emergency surgery (p = 0.02). There was however no reduction in mortality (23).

Swain et al have present preliminary data from an ongoing controlled trial of Nd:YAG photocoagulation in bleeding peptic ulcers. Of those who had bled from ulcers with visible vessels, 3 of the 17 in the treated group rebled compared with 12 of the 20 controls (p <0.025) (24).

CONCLUSIONS

The clinical experience obtained to date has shown that the risk of visceral perforation is minimal with this laser when correct energy levels are used but there does appear to be an increased risk when photocoagulation is repeated (7).

To date, it has been shown that the occurrence of further hemorrhage and the need for emergency surgery has been reduced, but the results from further controlled trials are awaited to see if these findings can be confirmed. There is as yet, no evidence that the mortality from peptic ulcer hemorrhage can be reduced and larger numbers of patients will have to be treated to determine this.

Laser photocoagulation has limitations in that it is apparent that the patient who has massive arterial hemorrhage at the time of endoscopy should be submitted to surgery immediately (23). There are patients who cannot be treated because of inaccessibility of the ulcer; for example, in a distorted, narrow duodenal bulb, or when the ulcer is very high up on the lesser curve of the stomach (22,23,24). There are patients in whom laser photocoagulation produces initial hemostasis and bleeding recurs. Information is required on the optimal parameters of radiation to be used and the actual technique of photocoagulation (22).

It remains unclear as to the maximum size of vessels that can be photocoagulated successfully and this depends to a large extent on the individual interpretation of what a vessel or artery is. It is therefore necessary to standardize the visual appearances of a vessel and an artery and to record whether it is actively bleeding or not before true comparisons between different series can be made.

Now that the patient who has a high risk of rebleeding can be identified at endoscopy, selective early surgery can be done with a probable reduction in post-operative mortality. It is against this that the true efficacy of Neodymium YAG photocoagulation must be judged.

REFERENCES

1. Allan R, Dykes P. (1976) Journal of Medicine, 45, 533-550.
2. Jones FA. (1956) Gastroenterology, 30, 166-190.
3. Johnston SJ, et al. (1973) British Medical Journal, iii, 655-660.
4. Dronfield MW. (1979) Journal of the Royal College of Physicians,
    London, 13, 84-86.
5. Cotton PB, et al. (1973) British Medical Journal, 2, 505-509.
6. Gilbert DA, Silverstein FE, Tedesco FS, et al. (1981) American Journal
    of Digestive Diseases, 26, 555-595.
7. Kiefhaber P, Nath G, Moritz K. (1977) Progress in Surgery, 15, 140-155.
8. Hillenkamp F. (1980) In Hillenkamp F, Pratesi R, and Sacchi CA, Lasers
    in Medicine and Biology. New York, Plenum Press, 39-68.
9. Longini RL, Zdrojkowski R. (1968) Trans. Biomed. Eng., 15, 4-10.
10. Halldorsson T, Langerhole J. (1978) Applied Optics, 17, 39-48.
11. Silverstein FE, Protell RL, Gilbert DA, et al. (1979) Gastroenterology,
    77, 491-496.
12. Dixon JA, Berenson MM, McLoskey DW. (1979) Gastroenterology, 77,
    647-651.
13. Brown SG, Salmon PR, Storey DW, et al. (1981) Gut, 21, 818-825.
14. Rutgeerts P, et al. (1981) Gut, 22, 38-44.
15. Hurst AF, Stewart MJ. (1929) In Gastric and duodenal ulcer. Oxford
    University Press, 76-132.
16. Griffiths WJ, Neumaun DA, Welsh JD. (1979) New England Journal of
    Medicine, 300, 1411-1413.
17. Dennis MB, et al. (1981) Gastroenterology, 80, 1522-1527.
18. Kicfhaber P, et al. (1979) 3rd International Congress for Laser Surgery.
    Graz, Austria.
19. Gulacsik C, Auth DC, and Silverstein FE. (1979) Applied Optics, 18,
    1816-1823.
20. Macleod IA, Bow CR, Joffe SN. (1982) Endoscopy, 14, 9-10.
21. Ihre T, Johansson C, Seligson U, and Torngren S. (1981) Scandanavian
    Journal of Gastroenterology, 16, 633-640.
22. Rutgeerts P, Vantrappen G, Broechaert L, et al. (1982) Gastroenterology,
    83, 410-416.
23. Macleod IA, et al. (1983) British Medical Journal, 286, 345-348.
24. Swain CP, et al. (1982) Gut.

CHAPTER 5

USE OF THE Nd:YAG LASER IN THE TREATMENT

OF NON-BLEEDING G.I. LESIONS

PRINCIPAL AUTHOR:

J.M. Brunetaud
Centre Multidisciplinaire traitement par laser
  and Clinique des maladies de l'appareil digestif
Hôpital Régional
59037 Lille Cedex
France

USE OF THE ND YAG LASER IN THE TREATMENT OF NON BLEEDING G.I. LESIONS.

J.M. BRUNETAUD, L. MOSQUET.
Centre Multidisciplinaire de traitement par laser and Clinique des maladies de l'appareil digestif, Hôpital Régional, 59037 Lille Cedex France.

INTRODUCTION

The first applications of lasers in digestive endoscopy were the treatment of hemorrhagic lesions . Since 1977, when we started to use lasers, efficacy and safety in these indications have been widely proven. Several non bleeding G.I. lesions can also be treated by lasers, with a considerable improvement compared to conventional treatment. We will report our experience on 89 patients in 2 kinds of indications : rectal villous adenomas, and palliative treatment of digestive cancers.

INSTRUMENTS

1- The lasers
    Our multidisciplinary center is equipped with several lasers. Two are currently used in digestive endoscopy : argon and Nd : YAG lasers. They are commercial products but probes and hand-pieces are prototypes manufactured by our technical research institute.
    The argon laser is the COOPER 770 (California USA) whose maximal output is 10 Watts. The Nd. YAG is the YAG MEDICAL 100 CILAS Biophysic Medical (France) ; the maximal output varies with the exposure time, from 120 Watts for 0.2 sec., to 80 Watts for 0.7 sec. and over 50 Watts in continuous mode.

2- The fibers
    All our optical fibers are produced by Fibres Optiques Industries, France. We use the 200/250 type argon and the 400/500 type for Nd. YAG. In digestive endoscopy, the fiber is wrapped into a teflon catheter (laser probe) ; for external use, the fiber is coupled to a hand piece, sort of pencil with 3 different types of lens.
    For argon, the laser probe has an external diameter of 1.7 mm and can be introduced in every type of forward or side viewing endoscopes. The hand piece can give 3 spots : 0.2, 0.6 and 1.2 mm. External diameter of Nd.: YAG laser probe is also 1.7 mm and fits for forward viewing endo-scopes, including pediatric model. The spot diameters given by the hand piece are 0.4, 1 and 2 mm. The very small size of our laser probes (1.7 mm compared to 2.2 mm for commercial products) allow the exhaustion of gas through the biopsy channel of conventional endoscope (inner diameter 2.8 mm) ; this is very helpful for upper G.I. endoscopy to avoid over dis-tension and pain.

3- Choice of the laser
    In our experience we must have the argon and Nd. YAG lasers available at the same time in the endoscopy room.The choice depends on the penetra-tion of the wavelength. For superficial lesions we use the argon, for deeper ones the Nd. YAG. In many cases we use both on the same patient (1).

A- RECTAL VILLOUS ADENOMAS

1- Technique
    Up to a distance of 10 cm from the anus, lesions can be treated under

rigid endoscopy through the hand-piece. This technique permits aspiration of secretions, blood, and necrosed tissue through a large canula. Beyond 10 cm, a rectosigmoïdoscope (Olympus ITS2) is used with the laser probe. A flexible canula (gastric aspiration tube Charrière N° 18) is introduced in the anus alongside the endoscope to ventilate the gas. The other tip of the canula is into a 2 liters bottle of water, in order to maintain a permanent pressure in the rectum (equal to the height of liquid).

2- Method
Despite multiple biopsies, any conservative treatment does not allow to obtain a complete histologic study of the lesion. In the particular case of villous adenomas, which is considered by many authors as a premalignant tumor, we have only treated patients with no signs of malignancy on multiple biopsies. They were all outpatients and they just received a small enema before endoscopy. The cure starts at a rhythm of 3 sessions a week until complete destruction of the tumor is obtained. After the initial destruction of the tumor, controls are performed once a week until complete cicatrisation with normal mucosa at endoscopy and histology and then every three months.

3- Patients
The 37 patients were 16 males an 21 females, and their average age was 70. Twenty-one patients were treated for the first time ; for 12 of them, a reduction of the tumoral volume was obtained by diathermic resection before laser. The other 16 patients had a recurrence after a conventionnal treatment : surgery (4), surgery + X-ray therapy (4), diathermic resection (8). The average time between the initial treatment and laser treatment was 2 years (2 months to 5 years). All the lesions were sessile and for 11 patients the tumor covered more than 3/4 of the rectum circumference.

4- Results
Symptoms disappear when a 3/4 tumoral volume reduction is obtained and patient's condition is always considerably improved . Patients are considered as cured when, 3 months after the last treatment, there are no macroscopic and histologic signs of recurrency. Among the 37 patients, 27 are cured with an average follow up of 8.3 months (3 to 24 months). In 5 patients the biopsies performed during the treatment have revealed an invasive carcinoma. Three had surgery without any sign of malignancy on the resected specimen. For the 2 others, the laser treatment was continued, as a palliative treatment. In 2 cases, laser treatment appeared inefficient : the tumor was regrowing at the same place after destruction. The last 3 patients were not able to be followed up.
No accidents occurred. In some instances, the treatment may be painful, especially when applied on area near to the anus. Minimal oozing often occurs during the 2 or 3 days after treatment ; 2 patients had a moderate hemorrhage (one during the treatment and one 3 days later), but no transfusion was required. Two patients who had a circumferential tumor developed a stenosis without symptoms. No rectal incontinence, perforation or fistula occurred (6).

5- Discussion
We have only treated a small number of patients and the follow up is short. However, this study allows some remarks :
- This method is efficient : 27 successes out of the 29 followed patients with no histological problems ;
- Treatment duration may be long in large lesions (up to 3 months) but it is performed without hospitalization ;
- The laser is effective on recurrences from one or more previous conventional treatments;

38

- Furthermore, it has not the side effects of other conservative methods like X-ray therapy or monopolar diathermy (hemorrhage, delayed cicatrisation, rectitis...).

B- PALLIATIVE TREATMENT OF DIGESTIVE CANCERS

If the laser is used for its thermal effects, the treatment of digestive cancers can only be considered as palliative. When treating a lesion from the mucosal side, we have no means to assess the depth of invasion. Photochemical treatment with hematoporphyrin derivatives or other substances may potentially have a more specific effect on malignant tissue but we so far have no clinical exprience (7).

1- Technique, method, patients

Nd. YAG laser is preferred to argon because of its better hemostatic effect and its deeper action. Not all patients with obstruction or hemorrhage can tolerate surgery. Therefore treatment frequency depends on the functional benefit ; at the beginning, they have laser twice or three times a week, and after improvement once a month. Different lesions and indications are reported on table II.

Location	Nb. patients	Indication
Oesophagus	8	Dysphagia-hemorrhages
Cardia	11	Dysphagia
Stomach	7	Hemorrhage
Duodenum	1	Stricture
Rectum	25	Rectorrhage-rectal syndrome
TOTAL = 52		

TABLE II : Digestive cancers and indication of laser treatments.

2- Results, discussion

Functional improvement is obtained after 1 or 2 weeks. Signs of obstruction are relieved and palliative surgery (gastrostomy or colostomy) is avoided. Bleeding slows down and number of blood transfusions is decreased. We cannot appreciate if laser treatment increases survival length but patient's comfort is certainly improved. In 3 cases the treatment has perhaps been curative : 1 gastric and 2 rectal carcinomas with a follow up of 6,4 and 10 months. In these 3 cases the lesions were small, less than 2 cm in diameter. Our results as palliative therapy are similar to those generally published by western authors (2). Japanese are testing the curative effect of the lasers in "early gastric cancers" which is a completely different disease from the western superficial gastric cancer (3, 4).

The 89 cases of rectal villous adenomas and digestive cancers are a small part of our 326 patients treated since July 1977 (5) which includes 141 acute hemorrhages, 32 angiomas and 64 other non- bleeding digestive lesions : 25 polyposis, 7 biliary and pancreatic cyst and 32 anal condylom. For the latter we only use argon laser.

REFERENCES

1. BRUNETAUD J.M., BISERTE J., CHARLIER J., LAFFITTE J.J., ROTTELEUR G., VANDENBUSSCHE P., BOUREZ J. Therapeutic applications of argon ion and Nd.Yag lasers. Laser TOKYO' 1981.

2. FLEISCHER D., KESSLER F., HAYE O. Endoscopic Nd. YAG laser therapy carcinoma of the oesophagus : a palliative approach. Am. J. Surg., 1982, 143, 280-283.

3. ITO Y., SUGIURA H., KIRAOKA Y., KASUGAI T. Endoscopic laser treatment of bordeline lesions and early gastric carcinomas. Laser TOKYO'1980.

4. MIZUSHIMA K., KARADA K., NAMIKI M., KASAI S., MITO M. Endoscopic therapy of the YAG laser in early gastric cancer and gastric polyps. Laser TOKYO'1980.

5. MOSQUET L. Le laser en gastro-entérologie : étude clinique sur 251 malades. Thèse, Lille 1982.

6. MOSQUET L., BRUNETAUD J.M. CORTOT A., BOUREZ J., HOUCKE M., DELMOTTE J.J., PARIS J.C. Le traitement endoscopic par laser des tumeurs villeuses rectosigmoïdiennes : résultats préliminaires. Gastro Enterol. Clin. Biol., 1983, 7, 60A (Abstract).

7. PATRICE T. Expérience Nantaise de l'utilisation du laser dans la destruction des tumeurs cliniques et expérimentales. Thèse, Nantes, 1981.

CHAPTER 6

ENDOSCOPIC Nd:YAG LASER THERAPY FOR DISEASES OF THE ESOPHAGUS

David E. Fleischer, M.D.
Cleveland Clinic Foundation
Cleveland, Ohio

Endoscopic Nd:YAG Laser Therapy for Diseases of the Esophagus
David Fleischer, M.D. Cleveland Clinic Foundation

INTRODUCTION

Endoscopic Nd:YAG laser therapy has been used to treat both bleeding and obstructing lesions of the esophagus. Laser treatment for bleeding Mallory-Weiss tears is universally performed by those who use laser therapy for gastrointestinal bleeding. A smaller percentage of those physicians use the laser for variceal bleeding and although some investigators have a substantial experience, the actual number is declining as the use of injection sclerotherapy increases. Endoscopic therapy of esophageal neoplasms, which is generally applied for palliation, has added a promising new dimension to the therapeutic armamentarium for a disease with a very grave prognosis. There are isolated. reports of esophageal webs and benign strictures being treated by endoscopic laser therapy.

Esophageal Bleeding

Conceptually variceal bleeding differs from most other types of gastrointestinal hemorrhage. It is venous bleeding and the vessels are generally visible and dilated without circumferential tissue support. And it is generally a secondary event (caused by portal hypertension and often underlying hepatic disease) as opposed to the primary nature of an ulcer bleed. Therefore control of the hemorrhage may be an important medical intervention at a given instant, but it does little to alter the primary underlying disease. And so for whatever unknown reason that bleeding developed, it is likely to occur again. And even though variceal sclerosis does not alter the underlying liver disease, it does alter the anatomic structure of the variceal columns in a way that could possibly reduce the likelihood of rebleeding.

Some, predominatly European, investigators have employed laser therapy for acute variceal bleeding. Kiefhaber[1] has treated more than one hundred patients with acute variceal bleeding with success in obtaining initial hemostasis in approximately 90% of cases. The results of Schonekas[2] and Sander[3] in other large series are equally impressive. Kiefhaber has now begun to employ sclerotherapy for long term management of varices after initial laser hemostasis.

Fleischer[4] has published the only randomized controlled study using Nd:YAG laser therapy for active variceal bleeding. Twenty patients whose variceal bleeding was persistent (red blood per NG tube/ 4 hours) and severe (> 2 units blood transfusion /4 hours or orthostasis 2° to blood loss) were included. Management was carried out by two teams of physicians. Team A made management decisions but did not know the nature of the endoscopic intervention (i.e. laser vs. sham treatment). Ten patients were randomized to each group. Age, etiology of varices, Child's classification, and other prognostic indicators were similar in both groups. Immediate hemostasis was achieved in seven of the ten patients in the laser group. No patients in the sham group stopped spontaneously, but four stopped with intravenous pitressin. However 7 of 10 in each group had either rebleeding or continued bleeding which necessitated a more definitive intervention (Sengstaken tube, transhepatic embolization, shunt or sclerotherapy). Blood transfusion requirements were similar in the two groups. Four laser treated and six sham-treated died during the hospitalization. In this study, laser therapy was more effective than sham treatment for initial therapy but did not alter the outcome. It is conceivable that laser therapy could have a role in attempts to achieve initial hemostasis, but if it is to play a major role in therapy, it must be followed by a more definitive treatment.

Bleeding from Mallory-Weiss tears is generally self-limited[5,6]. However some patient with this condition continue to bleed. Although there are no reports of laser therapy for bleeding Mallory-Weiss lesions per se, most investigators have had good success treating this lesion. Two large

Neodymium-YAG Laser in Medicine and Surgery, Joffe, Muckerheide, and Goldman, editors

series[1,7] number Mallory-Weiss patients among those included in their patient population.

Esophageal Obstruction

By varying the temperature deposited at a given site, the tissue effect
may be either coagulation (which is seen with temperatures in the range of
60°C) or vaporization (temperature > 100°C). Vaporization would be an undes-
ired effect in the treatment of bleeding (it contributes to laser-induced
bleeding), but it is a very desirable characteristic for the destruction of
an obstructing esophageal lesion such as a neoplasm.
Endoscopic management of esophageal cancer has several appealing aspects: 1) It averts the need for surgery and general anesthesia with their
attendant morbidity; 2) It diminishes considerably the likelihood of systemic side effects; 3) It can be performed under direct vision; 4) Unlike
radiotherapy, there is no maximum dose, so that if the tumor recurs in the
same area, re-treatment can be performed. It is limited in that it does not
affect pathologic tissue outside the gastrointestinal lumen and in that regard it is generally palliative.
Since the fiberoptic endoscope can place the physician in close proximity to neoplasms in the esophagus, stomach, and proximal duodenum, an opportunity exists for local oncolytic therapy. If laser energy is delivered
in such a fashion as to cause tissue vaporization and ablation, destruction
of tumor tissue can occur.
The first animal work using lasers to destroy neoplasms was done in the
1960s using a variety of lasers. In 1963, McGuff et al.[8-10] demonstrated
that ruby laser could destroy solid hepatic metastatic nodules. He also
treated methylcholanthrene-induced fibrosarcomas and malignant melanomas in
hamsters. In 1964, Minton and co-workers[11,12] described the use of the Nd
laser to destroy melanomas, sarcomas and mammary adenocarcinoma in animals.
Minton et al. used a Nd laser to treat multiple intraabdominal implants in
rabbits[13] and melanomas and sarcomas in mice[14]. Mullins et al.[15] destroyed
chemically induced primate hepatomas with the Nd laser. When Ketcham et al[16]
reviewed the role of the laser in cancer they predicted that it would
likely become an integral part of many biomedical laboratories because of its
ability to destroy selected components of the living cell.
Esophageal carcinoma is often diagnosed by endoscopy. Of the potentially curvative treatments, surgery and radiotherapy are the two most commonly employed. Unfortunately, it is far more common for the treatment of
esophageal cancer to be palliative rather than curative.
Currently existing methods of palliation for esophageal cancer include
surgery, radiotherapy, bougienage, prosthetic stents, and gastrostomy or
pharyngostomy. More recently, chemotherapy has been used. These are employed to relieve symptoms of dysphagia, odynophagia, chest pain, or bleeding.
Each of the palliative modalities may be of benefit in selected cases, but
each carries specific limitations. Surgery may not be technically feasible
because of the location of the tumor and the condition of the patient. In
addition, it has a well-recognized morbidity and mortality. Radiation therapy may take several weeks to provide symptomatic relief and if a recurrence
develops after the patient has received a maximal dosage it cannot be re-
employed. The attendant side effects of nausea, ill-feeling and potential
damage to organs outside the esophagus are still problematic. These latter
side effects exist as well with chemotherapy. It is too early to assess the
efficacy and safety of chemotherapy because the data is just emerging. Bougienage, with or without the placement of prosthetic stents, has provided
symptomatic benefit in certain patients[17-19]. In some patients, the strictured area is too small to allow clinically important dilatation. In others,
the tumor distortion makes dilatation difficult or impossible. Complications
may accompany these procedures (e.g. perforation, bleeding). Additionally, since tumor is 'stretched' rather than destroyed, repeated dilatations
are generally necessary. Pharyngostomy or gastrostomy open an avenue through

which nutrition can be poured into the gastrointestinal tract but they de-
prive the patient of the pleasure of ingesting food and have limited patient
appeal. For these reasons, any new form of palliation that may be effective
should be studied critically to determine its efficacy and safety.

The largest published series by Fleischer[20] describes 14 patients who
were not candidates for curative resection. The following selection criteria were used:

a. Patients with biopsy proven squamous cell carcinoma.
b. In whom it was unanimously agreed upon by the Departments of Surgery, Radiotherapy, Oncology, and Gastroenterology that no curative
   treatment was possible.
c. Who were not surgical candidates (i.e. disease in proximal half of
   esophagus), and
d. Who either developed a recurrence after previous radiotherapy or
   who were deemed to be better laser candidates than radiotherapy
   candidates by a joint agreement of both the Radiation Therapy and
   Gastroenterology Departments on basis of need for rapid relief of
   obstruction, overall clinical status, ability to undergo a course
   of radiation, and nutritional status. Therefore, it should be understood that in this patient population that no curative treatment
   existed or that if one did exist it was felt to have specific limitations in the patient under consideration. In this study, esophageal dilatation was employed only as an adjunct after laser therapy.

This technique is described as follows: Endoscopic laser therapy was
carried out in a conventional endoscopic suite using an Nd:YAG laser (Molectron) with a power output of 30 to 100 watts. The laser energy was conveyed
by way of a quartz waveguide through the biopsy channel of a therapeutic endoscope (Olympus GIF-1T or Olympus GIF-2T). Laser treatment was carried out
under direct vision. Patients were prepared with a topical anesthetic and
sedated with meperidine and diazepam.

The initial treatment is directed circumferentially around the luminal
opening, widening the circle toward the esophageal wall. (Fig. 1)

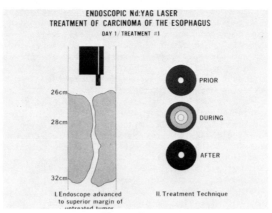

Figure 1.

The first tissue reaction is a white circular burn where the beam hits
the tumor tissue. If the laser beam is continuously focused on the same
site, cavitation occurs if the tip of the fiber is close (less than 1 cm to
the tissue) and the energy is high (70 to 90 watts). At times bleeding occurs and a black charred appearance develops when the Nd:YAG beam hits the
bloody tissue. Treatment continues until the superior margin of the tumor
has been treated. (Fig.2)

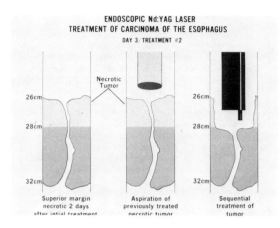

ENDOSCOPIC Nd:YAG LASER
TREATMENT OF CARCINOMA OF THE ESOPHAGUS
DAY 3/TREATMENT #2

| Superior margin necrotic 2 days after intial treatment | Aspiration of previously treated necrotic tumor | Sequential treatment of tumor |

When the treated area is observed 48 hours later, the previously treated area is whitish-yellow, soft and necrotic. The destroyed tumor is evacuated with forceps, polyp grasper or aspiration. Treatment is then begun on the underlying, previously untreated tumor. Laser treatment is continued until the lumen is sufficiently opened to permit passage of the endoscope into the stomach. If necessary, dilatation with mercury dilators is performed.

Thirteen men and one woman ranging in age from 49-82 years (mean 60 years) were treated. Six of the 14 patients had already undergone radiotherapy so virtually no other treatment was even available save dilatation or gastrostomy and in several of the patients, esophageal dilation had already been attempted and either was unsuccessful or technically not possible. Therefore, it is worth stressing that this group of patients with squamous cell carcinoma is highly selected and the prognosis would be considered dismal by most physicians who are familiar with this condition.

The symptomatic benefit derived by the patients is outlined in Table I. All 14 patients improved with laser therapy. Ten of 14 were symptomatic after therapy.

The survival in this group of patients was generally 2 to 3 months. Many were still able to eat solid foods until their death. This short survival period should be put into the perspective of this patient population (i.e. several had exhausted all alternative therapies at the time laser treatment was instituted). The emphasis should be placed on quality of life after treatment. Most were able to leave the hospital and most were able to enjoy solid foods.

The gross and histologic appearances were typical of squamous cell carcinoma of the proximal and mid-esophagus. The tumors varied in length from 5 to 10 cm. Most caused significant luminal obstruction and typical symptoms.

The mean number of treatments required to obtain relief of obstruction was 5.3. With the exception of patient, J.K., the second patient treated, all patients had 7 or less treatment sessions. The mean time span for relief of less than 2 weeks (11.6 days) compares favorably with radiation therapy. Patients tolerated the treatments well. There were 74 individual treatment sessions in the 14 patients. Preparation was not different from routine upper pan endoscopy.

The mean energy delivered per treatment was 4615 w-sec. (Table II) and and the total energy per patient averaged 24, 394 w-sec with a range of 2592 - 70, 217 w-sec. The total energy used correlated with tumor length and degree of luminal obstruction.

Minor complications occurred in a few patients and major complications in 2. Six patients had either lowgrade temperature elevations (> 100°F) and /or mild leukocytosis (> 12,500/cm^3) after treatments. These are described as complications although it is presumed that these parameters reflect the tissue inflammation and destruction that accompanied the treatment. In no patient was sepsis apparent. Five patients had pain during 1 or more treatment sessions. This invariably was relieved with increased analgesia. In no patient was hemorrhage a problem.

Major complications occurred in 2 patients. Patient, J.J. developed a tracheo-esophageal fistula 1 week after the last laser treatment. He had a previous course of radiotherapy and some dilatation after his last laser treatment. Dilatation is frequently performed because it can debride tissue made necrotic by laser. Since tracheo-esophageal fistulae may occur in esophageal carcinoma that has not been treated at all and since it can occur as a complication of both radiotherapy or esophageal dilatation, the laser may not have been a factor in this patient. Nonetheless, the fistula developed after laser therapy and it must be considered as a possible contributing factor. The patient's fistula was successfully treated with a perorally placed esophageal prosthesis. Patient J.M. was being treated by a physician under the supervision of Dr. Fleischer. After the obstructed lumen had been opened by the laser, esophageal dilatation was being performed for purposes of debridement. Immediately after the dilatation the patient developed severe chest pain and a perforation was demonstrated on barium swallow. Surgery was required to drain fluid from the chest. Eventually the patient could swallow without problem. Again this complication occurred in association with the laser therapy, although it was the related procedure, dilatation, which appeared to precipitate the complication.

In addition to these initial fourteen patients treated by Fleischer which are reported in the literature, an additional twenty other (non-published) cases have been treated. Results are similar although more energy is usually given per session and mean numbers of treatments is four/patient. Bown[21] in London has also had encouraging experience with Nd:YAG laser therapy of esophageal carcinoma. A very important series of patients treated by Mellow[22] was presented recently. Not only were patients benefited by laser therapy, but when he compared his laser treated patients to a group of matched historical controls statistically significant benefit was demonstrated in the treated group with regard to symptom improvement, performance status, and survival.

It should be stressed that the overwhelming majority of cases have had palliation as the goal of therapy. However, isolated cases of curative treatment have been described (Cremer, personal communication).

In addition to malignant obstruction, some reports of laser therapy for benign esophageal obstruction have been reported. These include webs, peptic strictures, and obstruction caused by EEA stapling procedure at the anastomotic site.

Summary

As described, endoscopic Nd:YAG laser therapy has been used for the therapy of several esophageal diseases. A more prolonged period of follow-up will be needed to know where these treatment techniques will fit in the overall management of the diseases for which they have been applied as well as other diseases. Initial results are encouraging.

TABLE I

SYMPTOMS BEFORE AND AFTER LASER THERAPY

PATIENT	AGE	SEX	PREV R-T	DYSPHAGIA		ODYNOPHAGIA		CHEST PAIN	
				PRE	POST	PRE	POST	PRE	POST
WP	60	M	(-)	0	0	0	0	2	0
JK	60	M	(-)	3	1	0	0	0	0
MT	49	M	(-)	2	0	1	0	0	0
LA	64	M	(+)	1	0	1	0	0	0
EZ	59	M	(-)	3	0	0	0	0	0
JH	62	M	(+)	3	0	0	0	2	1
AR	64	M	(-)	0	0	1	0	1	0
CJ	50	M	(+)	1	0	0	0	0	0
MB	65	M	(-)	3	0	1	0	1	0
GL	60	M	(-)	2	0	1	0	0	0
JJ	58	M	(+)	2	0	0	0	3	1
JA	67	M	(+)	2	0	0	0	0	0
AD	82	F	(+)	3	0	1	0	0	0
JM	50	M	(-)	3	1	3	1	3	2

Grading of symptoms: Dysphagia: 0 = None; 1 - Eats solids, food occasionally sticks; 2 - Eats only liquids. Odynophagia and chest pain: 0 = None; 1 = Minimal pain, no analgesics; 2 = Moderate pain, occasional analgesics; 3 = Severe pain.

TABLE II

DETAILS OF ENDOSCOPIC LASER THERAPY

PATIENT	TUMOR EXTENT (cm)	TUMOR LENGTH (cm)	LUM. OCCLUS. (%)	NO. RXS	TIME SPAN (days)	ENERGY/ RX. mean (w-sec)	TOTAL ENERGY (w-sec)
WP	25-33	8	60	7	19	3867	27,069
JK	24-31	7	95	13	28	5401	70,217
MT	28-39	11	90	6	13	4769	28,614
LA	25-30	5	95	5	12	4825	24,125
EZ	27-33	6	95	4	8	6214	24,859
JH	28-39	11	25-80	4	7	3383	13,531
AR	29-37	8	20-90	3	5	5541	16,623
CJ	17-25	8	95	6	14	4419	26,519
MB	20-27	7	20-95	2	3	1296	2,592
GL	19-30	11	90	4	8	6493	25,972
JJ	26-34	8	95	4	7	5145	20,583
JA	30-35	5	85	3	7	4532	13,596
AD	20-29	9	95	7	18	3627	25,394
JM	27-38	11	90	6	14	5094	30,564

50

References

1. Kiefhaber, P.,Nath G., Moritz, K.: Endoscopic control of massive gastrointestinal hemorrhage by irradiation with a high power Nd:YAG laser. Prog.Surg. 15:140, 1977.
2. Sander, R., Posl, M., Spuhler, A., Hitzler, H. Der Neodymium-YAG-Laser: Ein effektives instrument for dic stillung lebensbedrohlichen gastro-intestinal blutungen. Leber Magen Darm. 11: 31, 1981.
3. Schonekas, European Survey Data, 1980.
4. Fleischer, D. Nd:YAG laser therapy for active variceal bleeding. Gastroenterology 82: 1058, 1982.
5. Knauer, MC, Mallory Weiss Syndrome. Gastroenterology 71:5, 1976
6. Graham, D.Y and Schwartz,J.T. The spectrum of the MW tear. Medicine 57:407, 1977.
7. Rutgeerts, P., VanTrappen, G., Broeckbart, L., et al. Controlled trial of YAG laser treatment for upper digestive hemorrhage. Gastroentero-logy 83:410, 1982.
8. McGuff, P., Bushnell, D., Soroff, H., et al. Studies of the surgical applications of laser. Surg. Forum 14:143, 1963.
9. McGuff, P., Deterling, R., Bushnell, D., Gottlieb, L., Roeber, F., Fahimi, M.D. Laser radiation of malignancies. Ann. N.Y. Acad. Sci. 122:747, 1965.
10. McGuff, P., Deterling, R., Gottlieb, L., Fahimi, M.D., Bushnell, D., Roeber, F. Effects of laser radiation on tumor transplants. Fed. Proc. 24:S-150, 1965.
11. Minton, J., Ketcham, A., Dearman, J. Tumoricidal factor in laser radiation. Surg. Forum 15:335, 1964.
12. Minton, J., Ketcham, A. The laser, a unique oncolytic entity. Am. J. Surg. 108:845, 1964.
13. Minton, J., Ketcham, A., Dearman, J., McKnight, W.B. The application of pulsed, high-energy laser radiation to multiple intraabdominal tumor implants in experimental animals. Surgery 58:12, 1965.
14. Minton, J., Ketcham, A., Dearman, J., McKnight, W.B. The effect of neodymium laser radiation on two experimental malignant tumor systems. Surgery Gynec. Obstet. 122:481, 1965.
15. Mullins, F., Hoye, R. Ketcham, A., et al. Studies in laser destruction of chemically induced primate hepatomas. Am. Surg. 33: 298, 1967.
16. Ketcham, A., Hoye, R., Riggle, G. The laser: its role in cancer. Surg. Clins N. Am. 47:1249, 1967.
17. Boyce, H.W., Jr. Non-surgical measure to relieve distress of late esophageal carcinoma. Geriatrics 28:97, 1973.
18. Peura, D.A., Heit, H.A., Johnson, L.F., Boyce, M.W. Esophageal prosthesis in cancer. Am. J. Dig. Dis. 23:796, 1978.
19. Heit, H.A., Johnson, L.F., Siegel, S.R., Boyce, M.W. Palliative dilation for dysphagia in esophageal carcinoma. Ann. Intern. Med. 89: 629, 1978.
20. Fleischer, D.E. Endoscopic palliative laser therapy for carcinoma of the esophagus. Gastroenterology (in press, 1983).
21. Bown, S. Endoscopic laser therapy of upper gastrointestinal carcinomas, in: Gastrointestinal Disease, ed. Fleischer, D.E., Jensen, D., Bright-Asare, P., Martinus-Nijhoff publishers, The Hague, 1983.
22. Mellow, M., Pinkas, M., Frank, J., Waxman, M., Avigar, M. Endoscopic therapy for esophageal carcinoma with Nd:YAG laser. Prospective evaluation of efficacy, complications, and survival. Gastrointest. Endosc. 29:165, 1983.

CHAPTER 7

TUMOUR THERAPY WITH THE Nd:YAG LASER

S.G. Bown, M.D.
University College Hospital
London, United Kingdom

TUMOUR THERAPY WITH THE Nd YAG LASER

S G BOWN
University College Hospital, Gower Street, London, U.K.

Treatment of benign and malignant tumours with the Nd:YAG laser is at a very early stage of development. It has been used in 2 ways: a) to coagulate and necrose small tumours in situ and b) to debulk larger tumours. The latter has proved of value in palliation of advanced obstructing cancers of the upper gastrointestinal tract and main bronchi as endoscopic recanalisation can be achieved as discussed in another chapter of this book. Nevertheless, the techniques involved are relatively crude and in both cases, the treatment parameters used are based on empirical observations. Relatively little is known of precisely what happens in normal or neoplastic tissue close to the treated surface in relation to the treatment parameters used either in the short or long term. Fortunately, this does not appear to have led to major problems to date following Nd YAG laser treatment, although lack of such knowledge may have contributed to severe complications after another form of bronchoscopic laser therapy (1). It is the purpose of this chapter to discuss ways in which the sophistication of Nd:YAG laser treatment might be improved to extend the range of situations in which it might be able to cure or offer useful palliation to patients with neoplastic disease.

The precise biological effect of the laser beam at each point depends on many different factors. The most important of these are the light intensity, the absorption characteristics of the tissue and the biological response to the absorbed energy. All these vary throughout any target organ, so treatment of a tumour will show a range of effects, depending on the distance from the light source and the local constitution within the tumour (proximity to vascular stroma, degree of necrosis, amount of fibrous tissue etc). These will be discussed initially under the headings of spectrum and distribution of effects and then in the context of treating tumours in patients.

Spectrum of Effects

The range of Nd:YAG laser effects on neoplastic tissue is considerable. It covers:
        Immediate vaporisation
        Necrosis with subsequent sloughing
        Necrosis stimulating an inflammatory response with later fibrosis
        Remaining viable tumour

The laser energy is absorbed as heat and the most important determinant at each point is the energy absorbed per unit volume. A large amount of energy causes immediate vaporisation. Slightly lower levels cause thermal necrosis with later sloughing. The rate at which the energy is put in (the power) is not so critical in this context, although if the power is low, some of the energy absorbed may be conducted away from the target area thermally, reducing the severity of the damage. At very low power, a state of dynamic equilibrium can be reached in which the rate at which heat is conducted away from the target spot is the same as the rate at which laser energy is delivered. The power level is of particular importance when the laser is used for haemostasis. The primary haemostatic mechanism is thermal contraction of the walls of the bleeding vessel and of the surrounding tissue and experiments from several groups have shown that this is most effective using a power of 60-90 W (2,3).

© 1983 by Elsevier Science Publishing Co., Inc.
Neodymium-YAG Laser in Medicine and Surgery, Joffe, Muckerheide, and Goldman, editors

53

At local energy levels below those which lead to sloughing and overlapping with the range required for haemostasis, the thermal insult to the
tissue stimulates a local inflammatory response which can be followed by
the laying down of fibrous tissue (4). Fig 1 illustrates the two main

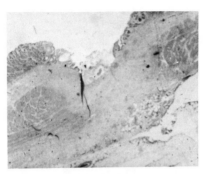

Fig 1: Normal canine stomach 2 weeks after laser treatment (375 J). The
mucosa has sloughed, but the submucosa and external muscle layer
have been replaced by dense fibrous tissue (H & E)

reactions to the laser in a section of canine stomach treated from the
mucosal side. The level exposed to the highest intensity (mucosa and part
of submucosa) has sloughed, whereas the lower intensity at the deeper
levels has stimulated an intense inflammatory response leading to replacement of muscle by fibrous tissue without perforation. A response of this
nature could replace parts of a tumour entirely by fibrous tissue although
nests of tumour cells could survive with the potential for further growth.
One study has even suggested that residual tumour may grow slightly more
rapidly after treatment than before although whether this is of
physiological significance has not been established (5). The mechanism of
thermal damage to cells (short of vaporisation) has not been firmly
established, but various possibilities have been suggested including
direct damage to DNA, membrane damage at the cell surface and lysozomes and
induction of special proteins (6). Collapse of the microvasculature may
also play a major part. This has been shown in recent work in dye laser
treatment of tumours by photoradiation therapy following sensitisation with
porphyrin derivatives, although in the latter case, the cytotoxic
mechanism is not thermal (7).

Malignant cells in general are probably no more sensitive to heat
than normal cells although sensitivity may be enhanced at low pH as might
be expected in the centre of tumours and certainly there are quantitative
differences between different cell lines (6). Even so, a similar range of
effects can be produced by the laser on normal tissue. Thus the key to
effective laser treatment must lie in delivering the appropriate energy to
neoplastic areas in such a way that the damage to adjacent normal tissue
does not exceed acceptable levels and that the tissue remaining at the
site of the tumour after therapy is able to maintain vital body functions
at all stages of the healing process. It is of no value to ablate a
gastric carcinoma and leave a large hole in the stomach wall. Achieving
the desired distribution of laser energy in relation to the anatomy of the
lesion being treated is the most difficult task in this whole approach to
tumour therapy, and is the aspect that has received least attention to
date from both experimental workers and clinicians.

Distribution of Effects

The distribution of biological effects depends on the light intensity at each point within a target organ. It is straightforward to determine the intensity on the surface immediately below an incident laser beam (although the amount that is reflected from the surface will vary with the angle of incidence and the optical properties of the surface). The intensity at all other points will depend on the optical properties of the organ, the most important of which are absorption and scattering. Near the surface absorption is dominant and the intensity falls as $1/r\, e^{-\alpha r}$ where r is the depth below the surface and α is the attenuation coefficient. At depths 2-3 times the scattering mean free path, the scattering becomes more important and the intensity falls as $1/r\, e^{-\alpha r}$ (8). However, in practice, formulae such as these can only give a rough approximation of likely intensities as all tissues, tumours particularly, are full of inhomogeneities which alter the attenuation coefficient and distort the pattern of light distribution. The best one can hope for is an estimate of the extent of the most important effects (necrosis with sloughing and necrosis followed by fibrosis) around each treatment point for given treatment parameters. For treatments aimed at debulking or recanalising obstructing tumours, high energy levels delivered to the area of maximum obstruction and kept away from the borders of the tumour are all that is required. If there is to be any prospect of ablating entire tumour masses, the most important zone is that where tumour necrosis is followed by fibrosis. This zone should be as wide as possible and must cover the region where neoplastic and normal tissue meet. This requires multiple carefully defined treatment points separated by distances which will depend on the extent of the zone of fibrosis for the treatment parameters used. For many tumours, only one surface is readily accessible (e.g. bronchial carcinoma at bronchoscopy). However, if the extent of tumour can be defined (e.g. by CAT scan) treatment is still theoretically possible using the interstitial technique. This was originally developed for transmitting the low power dye laser beam as required for photoradiation therapy with porphyrin sensitisation. The bare laser fibre is inserted directly into tissue instead of the conventional external approach of mounting the fibre in a thin plastic catheter which is held a short distance above the surface of the target organ. The technique is illustrated in Fig 2. There are several advantages. Treatment can be

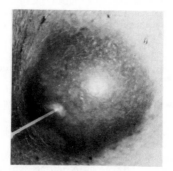

Fig 2: Interstitial technique. The bare laser fibre is inserted directly into the tumour mass (a cutaneous secondary deposit)

centred on any point within the tumour - the tip of the fibre acts as a point source and scattering produces a roughly spherical distribution of effects - and the treatment point can be carefully identified and the fibre fixed prior to transmission of the beam (more difficult with an external fibre). However, the fibre tip must be in contact with solid tissue at all times, so instant vaporisation is not possible which limits the maximum safe power. If a cavity develops around the tip, the delivered energy will not be conducted away and any debris on the tip will absorb the energy, which is likely to raise the temperature high enough to destroy the tip. An example of a skin secondary from a malignant melanoma treated by this means is shown in Fig 3. Close to the position where the fibre was inserted tumour has been replaced by fibrous tissue, whereas further out

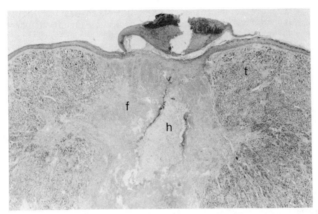

Fig 3: Cutaneous secondary deposit from a malignant melanoma 5 days after interstitial laser treatment. There is clear demarcation between the zones of fibrosis (f) and remaining viable tumour (t). The central hole (h) indicates the site of the fibre during treatment (H & E)

viable melanoma remains. It is likely that the use of a low laser power for a long exposure time will extend zone of fibrosis without putting the fibre at risk, but this will require careful assessment for each tumour type. More uniform illumination of a tumour mass can also be achieved using a diffuser tip to the fibre in which the light is emitted evenly in all directions from the last 1-2 cm instead of just the tip.

Once multiple treatment sites are used, many other questions arise and the most important of these concerns healing. The difference between necrosis with sloughing and necrosis followed by fibrosis will depend on the body's ability to produce an inflammatory response in that area as well as on the energy absorbed. Treatment of several immediately adjacent sites could impede the spread of capillaries and proliferation of fibroblasts in the most severely damaged areas. Safer, effective therapy might be carried out by spreading the treatment sites more initially and returning to treat the intermediate areas 1-2 weeks later. Another approach would be to treat multiple sites simultaneously, which would make the light intensity during therapy more uniform through the treated volume and would reduce the treatment time, although this has the disadvantage of treating adjacent areas at the same session. Only careful experiments can determine the relative merits of these various techniques.

The Nd YAG Laser in Context (11)

a) Alternative methods of achieving local hyperthermia

This laser provides local hyperthermia and first comparisons must be with other techniques for doing this. The Argon laser can provide similar precision, but tissue penetration is much less, which reduces the value for treating any lesion larger than a few millimetres in diameter. Three main non-laser approaches are currently under assessment and were recently reviewed in a supplement to the British Journal of Cancer (9). They are ultrasound, microwaves and radiofrequency induction heating. Superficial lesions are easy to treat by any of these modalities, but the problems arise trying to achieve local heating in internal organs. It is extremely difficult to localise the effects of any thermal treatment adequately by non-invasive applicators other than close to the skin and so invasive methods must be used. Microwaves can be transmitted with the aid of a radiating monopole (a miniature coaxial transmission line which can be made flexible and implanted surgically or via body orifices). Radiofrequency induction heating can be achieved by implanting ferromagnetic seeds (selectively heated by external inductive coils) or by using needle electrodes (10). The latter is essentially the same as diathermy, under which circumstances it is notoriously difficult to predict the energy dissipated and the distribution and extent of the effects produced. Nevertheless, the volume of tumour that can be usefully heated by these methods (radius 1-2 cm from the treatment point) is comparable to that heated with the Nd:YAG laser using the interstitial technique. Little work has yet been done on invasive, therapeutic ultrasound probes. However, ultrasound waves can be penetrating, directional and even focusable and they may have a role to play in this field in the future.

Until recently, lasers have not featured in most discussions of hyperthermia techniques. However, the ability to deliver energy in a precisely controlled manner to any position accessible to a single flexible fibre (inserted surgically or via a flexible endoscope) means that the precision of local heating with the Nd YAG laser is at least as good as, and probably superior to, any other current modality. In a recent review, Bleehan said "it is fair to say that no method (of hyperthermia) currently available permits an accuracy or versatility of treatment comparable with that possible with the ionising radiations used in radiotherapy" (6). Developments in laser technology may already be changing this situation.

b) Synergy with other therapeutic modalities

Synergy is possible with other techniques damaging tumour cells by non-thermal mechanisms. These include radiotherapy, chemotherapy and photoradiation therapy following sensitisation (e.g. with certain porphyrin derivatives). Heat and x-radiation act synergistically. Current experimental data suggests that similar effects of the combination are seen in normal and neoplastic tissue but that the time course is different. Experimental tumours recover more slowly than normal tissue and the therapeutic gain is greater when heat follows the x-radiation by several hours (6).

Local heat can be synergistic with various chemotherapeutic agents. It increases drug access with adriamycin and inhibits recovery from potentially lethal damage with bleomycin. Particular interest currently centres on the use of alkylating agents with heat for perfusion techniques (6).

Photoradiation therapy (PRT) is a new technique under assessment for selective tumour therapy. Certain porphyrin derivatives are retained longer in tumours than in normal tissue after systemic administration and following exposure to red light from a dye laser, act as sensitisers to produce singlet oxygen which at appropriate concentrations can kill cells (11). This is of particular interest as the same fibre delivery system might be used for the dye laser and for a Nd YAG laser enabling the same areas to be treated with each method and recent work suggests that PRT and hyperthermia may be synergistic (12).

Thus the Nd YAG laser is one of the most promising instruments for providing local hyperthermia. It may have a useful synergistic effect with other non-thermal methods such as radiotherapy and chemotherapy and does not have the cumulative toxicity problems of the latter two modalities.

Clinical Application

The clinical value of the Nd: YAG laser techniques described here in relation to alternative treatment modalities will depend on how predictable and reproducible the effects turn out to be and how wide the safety margin is to avoid unacceptable damage to adjacent tissue. Gardner et al (5) showed that in a subcutaneous tumour model in mice, the energy density required to eradicate tumours of a particular size by external Nd YAG irradiation is fairly constant and other reports have shown that the depth of tissue damage in normal tissue depends closely on the applied energy (3). Such quantitative results are difficult to obtain in man. Many small tumours in man have been treated with a view to cure on an empirical basis as described elsewhere in this book, but these are mainly in areas where the surrounding tissue can safely absorb large amounts of energy compared with that required to ablate the tumour. If full advantage is to be taken of the precision of control possible with the laser, careful quantitative studies must be carried out in animal tumours to relate the nature and extent of hyperthermic damage to the treatment parameters used in each situation.

Even with this knowledge, major problems remain. The situation is fast approaching when the precision possible for local hyperthermia exceeds the precision of localising the tumour by current diagnostic techniques (conventional radiology, computerised axial tomography, ultrasound, endoscopy etc). Unfortunately, no technique is sufficiently selective to make it possible to treat large volumes of normal tissue with impunity. Finally, the laser can only provide local therapy and has no role in the treatment of disseminated disease. Nevertheless, it provides an excellent means of ablating tumour tissue in a controlled manner and, under appropriate circumstances, replacing the neoplastic areas by fibrous tissue without loss of the mechanical integrity of the organ. Potentially, this is a major advance and deserves careful evaluation.

REFERENCES

1. Cortese D A, Kinsey J H. Endoscopic management of lung cancer with haematoporphyrin derivative phototherapy. Mayo Clinic Proceedings, 57, 543-7 (1982).
2. Rutgeerts P, Vantrappen G, Geboes K, Broeckaert L. Safety and efficacy of Neodymium YAG laser photocoagulation; an experimental study in dogs. Gut 22, 38-44 (1981).
3. Bown S G, Salmon P R, Storey D W et al. Nd YAG laser photocoagulation in the dog stomach. Gut 21, 818-25 (1980).
4. Kelly D F, Bown S G, Calder B M et al. Histological changes following Nd YAG laser photocoagulation in canine gastric mucosa. Gut 24 (1983).
5. Gardner W N, Hugh-Jones P, Carroll M A et al. Quantitative analysis of effect of Neodymium YAG laser on transplanted mouse carcinomas. Thorax 37, 594-7 (1982).
6. Bleehan N M. Hyperthermia in the treatment of cancer. Br. J. Cancer 45, Suppl V, 96-100 (1982).
7. Henderson B W, Dougherty T J. Studies on the mechanism of tumour destruction by photoradiation therapy. Proceedings of Clayton Foundation Symposium on Porphyrin Localisation and Treatment of Tumours. Plenum Press (in press) (1983).
8. Svaasand L O, Doiron D R, Profio A E. Light distribution in tissues during photoradiation therapy. Medical Imaging Science Group Report 900-01 (1981). University of California, Los Angeles.
9. British J. Cancer 45, Suppl V, (1982).
10. Cheung A Y. Microwave and radiofrequency techniques for clinical hyperthermia. Br. J. Cancer 45, Suppl V, 16-24 (1982).
11. Dougherty T J, Kaufman J E, Goldforb A et al. Photoradiation therapy for the treatment of malignant tumours. Cancer Res. 38, 2628-35 (1978).
12. Dougherty T J. Recent advances in Photoradiation Therapy. Proceedings of Clayton Foundation Symposium on Porphyrin Localisation and Treatment of Tumours. Plenum Press (in press) (1983).

CHAPTER 8

REPORT OF 1000 LASER ENDOBRONCHIAL RESECTIONS

Principal Author:

J.F. Dumon, M.D.
Dept. of Endoscopy
Salvator Hospital BP 51
13227 Marseille Cedex 2-France

60

REPORT OF 1000 YAG LASER ENDOBRONCHIAL RESECTIONS

DUMON J.F., MD., BOURCEREAU J., MD., MERIC B., MD.,JAHJAH F., MD., AUCOMTE
F., MD., DUPIN B., MD.
Dept. of Endoscopy Salvator Hospital BP 51 13277 Marseille Cedex 2-France.
Phone (91) 74.29.89.

ABSTRACT

This report sums up the experience of the Endoscopy Department of
Salvator Hospital in Marseille (800 treatments) and that of the Thoracic
Surgery Department of Marie Lannelongue Hospital in Paris (200 treatments).
All patients were treated according to the same two techniques i.e. 77.5 %
under general anesthesia with spontaneous ventilation using an open tube
and 22.5 % under local anesthesia using a fiberscope. In all cases the
laser used was the CILAS YAG Medical 100. The main indications were
malignant, uncertain prognosis and benign tracheobronchial tumors, tracheal
stenosis and miscellaneous indications. Accidents were rare, no fatality
occurred, the main problem being hemorrhage.

INTRODUCTION

The list of biomedical applications of laser energy continues to grow
as research and development in the field advances. Transmission via fiber
optics was the breakthrough which opened the way to endoscopic laser
treatment. In the hands of a skilled endoscopist, the inherent dangers of
the technique can be minimized and it has thus obviated a number of a
procedures formerly used for a variety of tedious and disagreeable tasks.
Its greatest success, however, has come in bronchoscopy where it
constitutes a therapeutic modality for numerous heretofore untreatable
endobronchial lesions.

This report sums up the experience accumulated from 3 years of daily
laser use by two French endoscopy teams using the same technique and the
same apparatus (Hopital Salvator Marseille : 800 treatments, Hopital Marie
Lannelongue Paris : 200 treatments).

MATERIAL AND METHODS

The laser instrument used is a YAG Laser (YM 100 CILAS). It has a 1.06
micron wavelength which is transmitted through a 2.5 mm diameter flexible
quartz fiber coated with teflon and cooled by a continuous air flow. The
laser's power is adjustable between 10 and 100 watts and can be used on an
intermittent or continuous basis. The treatment is made either under local
anesthesia with a fiberscope or general anesthesia with spontaneous
ventilation via an open tube.

We performed 1000 endoscopic laser resections on 527 patients. The
indications which motivated these operations can be divided into three
groups i.e.
- tracheobronchial tumors (331 cases).
- tracheal stenosis (111 cases)
- miscellaneous indications such as removal of suture threads or tissue
embedded foreign bodies (85 cases).

There were 89 women and 438 men whose ages ranged from 9 months to 86
years with the overall male and female average being 64 years.

Neodymium-YAG Laser in Medicine and Surgery, Joffe, Muckerheide, and Goldman, editors

INDICATIONS	No PATIENTS	No SESSIONS	A.GENERAL	A.LOCAL
TRACHEOBRONCHIAL TUMORS	331	619	530	89
TRACHEAL STENOSIS	111	257	197	60
MISCELLANEOUS	85	124	48	76
TOTAL	527	1000	775	225

As can be calculated from the above table, only 22.5 % of all the treatments done were performed under local anesthesia. At 61 % the percentage of local anesthesias was considerably higher for miscellaneous indications. In the following pages the main indications, i.e. tracheo-bronchial tumors, tracheal stenosis, and miscellaneous conditions, will be discussed.

TRACHEOBRONCHIAL TUMORS

In this section we will deal successively with malignant tumors, tumors with uncertain prognosis and benign tumors.

1. MALIGNANT TUMORS

Most of the laser resections were carried out on this type of lesion. In inoperable cases the technique proved itself to be highly effective and deserves to be ranked as an invaluable weapon in the fight against cancer. It can be used in addition to or in lieu of surgery with adjuvant radio-, chemo- or immuno-therapy. Caution must however be exercised since malignant tumors have a high hemorrhagic potential. Accordingly the use of an open tube under general anesthesia is mandatory for malignant tumors. In all 503 sessions were performed on 280 patients suffering from malignant tumors. This averages out to 1.7 sessions per patient. The mean patient age was 63.9 years, i.e. 64.5 for women (37) and 63 for men (243).

PATHOLOGY	No PATIENTS	No TREATMENTS	A.GENERAL	A.LOCAL
SQUAMOUS CELL	211	388	329	59
ADENOCARCINOMA	45	63	60	3
INDIFFERENTIATED	21	49	46	3
RARE TUMORS	3	3	3	0
TOTAL	280	503	438	65

PATHOLOGY

Squamous cell carcinomas were the most frequent. There was an unusually high occurence of adenocarcinoma in women. The rare tumors include one epitheliosarcoma, one fibroleiomyosarcoma and one lymphoma. Histological type had no apparent incidence on the immediate results, which were good or excellent in 244 out of 280 patients. This gives an overall success rate of 87 % which in function of histological type can be broken down to 89 % for squamous cell, 86.7 % for adenocarcinomas and 66 % for small cell and indifferentiated tumors. Finally it should be noted that, for the 22 secondary cancers treated, the success rate was 90.9 %. Twelve of these secondary lesions originated from squamous cell tumors (esophagus 9, bladder 2, tongue 1) and ten from glandular tumors (kidney 4, thyroid 4, breast 3).

PATHOLOGY	No PATIENTS	EXCELLENT*	FAIR**	POOR
SQUAMOUS CELL	211	99	89	23
ADENOCARCINOMAS	45	22	17	6
INDIFFERENTIATED AND SMALL CELL CARCINOMAS	21	9	5	7
RARE TUMORS	3	3	0	0
TOTAL	280	133	111	36

* excellent : normal tracheal gauge at end of treatment
** fair : improved ventilation

LOCATION

Location had the greatest influence on results. Success was highest in the trachea and right main stem bronchus where the percentage of good or excellent results was 95 and 92.8 % respectively. In the left main stem bronchus and right upper and middle lobes, resection was successful over 75 % of the time. Conversely, in the left upper and lower lobes, failures slightly outnumbered successes (50 %). Laser resection is most useful when applied to recent obstructions in the trachea and main stem bronchi. Such indications are the best, firstly because they create life-threatening situations which can be immediately remedied by laser treatment and secondly because in these two regions the chances of success are the highest.

LONG TERM RESULTS

Long term results are obviously hard to assess. Local growth of a tumor in an airway can in many cases be contained by repeated laser treatment. Usually one treatment every four months is sufficient for strictly endoluminal tumors. For tumors involving external compression, recurrences are unfortunately quicker. Since laser treatment in cancer cases is rarely used alone, it is hard to assess the degree of responsibility of each treatment in survival. It is however interesting that, in all cases of strictly endoluminal tracheal tumors, the survival time exceeded 18 months. Obviously the primary goal of laser therapy is not to cure cancer but rather to increase the quality of survival.

2. TUMORS WITH UNCERTAIN PROGNOSIS

This is a general heading under which a diversity of entities, formerly called mildly malignant tumors, are lumped. Some like adenoid cystic carcinomas and spindle-cell tumors are seldom susceptible to surgical excision while others like carcinoids almost always are. In any case, whenever possible, surgery should be preferred over endoscopic resection. With these lesions there is always a possibility of an extra-bronchial extension and a constant danger of metastasis.

Such tumors are in fact rare. In 3 years of experience, we have only encountered 18 cases : 7 adenoid cystic carcinomas, 9 carcinoid tumors, 1 spindle cell tumor and 1 adamantinoma. The results of the 60 resections which they motivated are summed up in the following table :

HISTOLOGY	No PATIENTS	No TREATMENTS	A.GENERAL	A.LOCAL
ADENOID CYSTIC C.	7	24	24	0
CARCINOID	9	23	20	3
SPINDLE-CELL	1	12	3	9
ADAMANTINOMA	1	2	1	1
TOTAL	18	61	48	13

Repeated sessions were necessary for most of these tumors and, in the case involving the spindle-cell lesion, 9 sessions under local anesthesia and 3 under general anesthesia were needed. Two patients, a 47 year-old woman suffering from a tracheal cylindroma and a 28 year-old man with a carcinoid in the left upper lobe, received subsequent surgery. Two adenoid cystic carcinomas and one carcinoid were postoperative recurrences.

3. BENIGN TUMORS

These rare tumors are the only type for which laser resection is generally preferable over surgical excision. We have treated 33 benign tumors :

PATHOLOGY	No PATIENTS	No TREATMENTS	A.GENERAL	A.LOCAL
PAPILLOMA	6	9	9	0
LIPOMA	5	18	12	6
TUBERCULOSIS	5	7	7	0
ANGIOMA	4	4	2	2
CHONDROMA	3	4	4	0
MISCELLANEOUS*	10	13	10	3
TOTAL	33	55	44	11

* 2 hamartomas, 2 leiomyofibromas, 1 neurofibroma, 1 abrikossof, 2 amyloidosis, 1 botryoid tumor, 1 tr. br. osteoplastica.

Papillomas were the most frequent tumors in this group. In view of the danger of malignancy, a careful histological analysis should always be made.

PATHOLOGY	No PATIENTS	No TREATMENTS	A.GENERAL	A.LOCAL
MALIGNANT	280	503	438	65
UNCERTAIN PROGNOSIS	18	61	48	13
BEGNIN	33	55	44	11
TOTAL	331	619	530	89

TRACHEAL STENOSIS

Tracheal stenosis is a serious condition which quickly becomes life-threatening. Most patients need emergency treatment before any further therapy can be undertaken. Pulmonologists, E.N.T's, and chest surgeons all have their own approach to this grave pathology. The laser constitutes still another tool for its treatment. Tracheal stenosis calls for an open tube resection under general anesthesia. Only smaller tracheal granulomas are amenable to fiberscopic resection under local anesthesia. Also deserving to be mentioned is the fact that to treat stenosis the operator must dispose of a full 3 to 12 mm set of open tubes. Which tube is used depends on the type of stenosis, but in general resection starts with the smallest tube and procedes with progressively larger ones. With stenosis, the primary purpose of the initial Yag Nd laser resection is to restore patency and enable acceptable ventilation. Subsequent treatment depends on a number of factors which will be discussed in correlation to results further on.

In our experience tracheal stenosis motivated 257 endoscopic resections on 111 patients. These stenoses fell into two categories :
- genuine tracheal stenosis usually appearing as a complication to tracheal intubation during resuscitation.
- granuloma-related stenosis occurring after sleeve resection or as a complication to a tracheotomy or tracheostomy.

TYPE OF STENOSIS	No PATIENTS	No TREATMENTS	A.GENERAL	A.LOCAL
GENUINE STENOSIS	62	163	155	8
GRANULOMAS	41	71	26	45
GRANULOMAS AFTER SLEEVE RESECTION	8	23	16	7
TOTAL	111	257	197	60

1. GENUINE TRACHEAL STENOSIS

These stenoses stem from secondary lesions caused by intubations or tracheotomies performed in intensive care. There are three kinds of genuine tracheal stenosis :
- concentric stenosis
- bottle-neck stenosis
- atypical stenosis

TYPE OF STENOSIS	No PATIENTS	No TREATMENTS
CONCENTRIC	11	19
BOTTLE-NECK	41	123
ATYPICAL	10	21
TOTAL	62	163

CONCENTRIC STENOSIS (11 cases)

This type of stenosis which is due to a fibrous outgrowth of a circular inflammation constitutes the best indication for laser resection. Such strictures can be readily erradicated without hemorrhage. On the average two sessions per patient are required. In our experience 7 of the cases treated have been stable for over 16 months.

BOTTLE-NECK STENOSIS (41 cases)

This type of stenosis is the most difficult to treat. It usually involves an inflammatory effused wall with one or more "humps" and/or sagging of the cartilage lining into the lumen. For such afflictions laser treatment must be combined with instrumental dilatation. As these stenosis are highly prone to recurrence two factors, stability and number of sessions, must be taken into account in evaluating the results.

Number of sessions In our initial attempts to apply laser resection to bottle-neck strictures, we were, in an alarming number of cases, confronted with the problem of recurrence and repeated treatments were needed. Indeed more than 5 laser sessions had to be performed on each of 5 patients all of whom suffered from highly inflammatory stenosis. Presently we are able to manage these stenos s in the first or second session by using a Montgomery tube. Not counting the aforesaid cases, the average number of sessions was 2 per patient.

Stability of results Twenty patients continue to show stationary results after over 6 months. For 8 patients a Montgomery tube was inserted during the endoscopic treatment. In 4 of these cases, the tubes have now been removed and the airways are clear. For 7 patients stenosis was definitively remedied by sleeve resection, however, this required up to 4 laser treatments for the airflow to be restored and surgery performed under good conditions. Of the remaining cases, 7 are very recent; 2 of foreign origin (Denmark and Italy) have been lost from sight; and one died from chronic respiratory insufficiency after a remission of three months.

ATYPICAL STENOSIS

Sprawling stenosis In four cases the stenosis covered a 3 cm long section of the trachea. The first was located just below the vocal cords, the second below the stoma and the third, a two-humped irregularity, at the bottom of the trachea. The first was treated by laser therapy alone and has been stable for 14 months. In the other three cases a Montgomery tube was used in addition to the laser. After removal of the tube, results were satisfactory in one case but the other case required sleeve resection.

Total stenosis Six patients all of whom had been tracheotomized for an extended period in intensive care presented well organized fibrotic occlusions just below the stoma. All six received a Montgomery tube. The oldest tube was removed 12 months ago but contact has been lost with the patient.

2. GRANULOMA-RELATED STENOSIS (49 CASES)

Symptomwise the distinction between tracheal granuloma and stenosis is not always clear especially when the granuloma occurs at the rim of a tracheotomy tube. They have been classified separately because treatment-wise they are quite different.

GRANULOMAS ON SUTURES AFTER SLEEVE RESECTION (8 CASES)

Some were quite large and, in extreme cases, caused subtotal occlusion of the tracheal lumen.

SOLITARY TRACHEAL GRANULOMAS (41 CASES)

1) granulomas and tracheotomy (29 cases) Laser resection was performed on 29 tracheotomized patients displaying granulomas at three different locations : ostial (8 cases), sub ostial (14 cases) supra ostial (7 cases).

2) granulomas in closed trachea (12 cases) Granulomas can occur for various reasons, after removal of a tracheotomy tube (6 cases), after intubation during intensive care (4 cases) or surgery on trachea (2 cases). In most cases isolated tracheal granulomas can be treated safely under local anesthesia with good or excellent results. Recurrence is rare.

MISCELLANEOUS APPLICATIONS

In addition to the applications heretofore described, the laser can be used endoscopically for a variety of smaller tasks. In most cases, a fiberscope and a local anesthesia can be safely used and the "heavy" technique is seldom necessary. These applications are either post-operative or medical.

1. POST-OPERATIVE APPLICATIONS

GRANULOMAS

A frequent and ideal use for the laser is the resection of post-operative granulomas which may appear on a suture thread months or even years after an operation. When a post-operative patient presents an irritative cough often accompanied by bleeding, a granuloma is to be suspected and an endoscopic inspection should be made. Usually these benign lesions have a smooth round surface and a wide base. In some cases they are elongated and are often congruent with suture threads. They can however have a more sinister malignant appearance, with budding and hemorrhagic aspects. A biopsy should always be made prior to resection to ascertain the benignancy of the lesion since histological study is no longer possible after resection. Once positive identification has been made, the laser can be efficiently used not only to destroy the granuloma but also, if necessary, to remove the offending suture. Bronchial fistula is a post-operative risk especially since it is hard to control the depth of the laser's action and it is obviously dangerous to cut a suture thread on a stump left after pneumonectomy.

SUTURE THREADS

Sometimes endoscopic inspection reveals that patients presenting symptoms of granuloma actually suffer from a suture thread which has worked its way out into the lumen. The laser can also be used in such cases provided that more than two weeks have elapsed since the operation. The procedure is quite simple. The suture thread is pulled out away frow the airway wall then the laser is positioned close to the thread near a point of entry and 1 or 2 half second shots at 35 or 40 watts are fired.The suture thread is thus cut and can be removed with a pair of forceps.

BRONCHIAL FISTULAS

Bronchial fistulas are rare lesions. Treatment is difficult,the standard protocol calls for proper drainage of the post pneumonectomy cavity, and endoscopic purging of the fistulized zone followed by regularly repeated nitratage. The laser can be of great service in this treatment for it can be used to get rid of suture threads and to clean the edges of the fistula opening. Nitratage should be conducted daily for 15 to 30 days. The laser can also be used to dislodge and remove suture threads or clips. A local anesthesia is usually sufficient but great care must be exercised in the proximity of vascular ligatures.

BRONCHIAL STENOSIS

Bronchial stenosis whether it be of surgical or infectious origin is seldom easy to manage. The laser has not proved to be any more expedient than other methods.

2. MEDICAL APPLICATIONS

TRACHEOBRONCHIAL HEMORRHAGES

Tracheobronchial hemorrhages are rare. They may however occur as in tracheotomized patients after a traumatic aspiration or biopsy. When classic methods fail, the laser is theoretically a simple means of coagulation. Obviously the laser can not be used for massive tuberculosis or radiotherapy-related hemorrhages.

TISSUE-EMBEDDED FOREIGN BODIES

On rare occasions, an attainable foreign body resists removal with conventional endoscopic tools. This can happen either because a granuloma is in the way or because of impactation . In the first case, the laser may be used to destroy the granuloma, and in the second, it can be used either to burn the foreign body out or to carve a "handle" on it.

The following table sums up the miscellaneous applications for which the laser was used.

(85) MISCELLANEOUS APPLICATIONS

SUTURE THREAD	44 (12 granulomas
GRANULOMAS	20
HEMORRHAGES	14
BRONCHIAL STENOSIS	4
FOREIGN BODY TISSUE EMBEDDED	3 (1 failure)

CASE REPORTS

Case 1 : A 58 year-old man was treated for a squamous cell carcinoma in the right main stem bronchus causing a total collapse of the right lung. In a single laser session, the passage was reopened and the airflow restored. His X-ray appeared normal. Radiotherapy was subsequently administered. His condition is stable after 7 months.

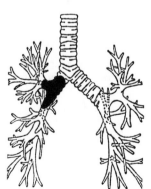
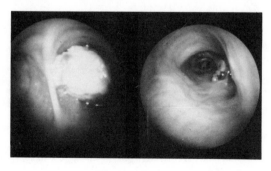

68

Case 2 : A tracheal papilloma was diagnosed in a 69 year-old woman in November 1980. The tumor was completely resected in one laser session. An endoscopic check-up 3 then 10 months later revealed no recurrence. Results have been stable for 17 months.

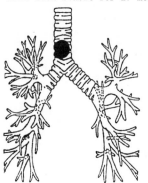 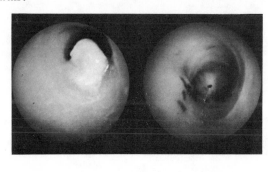

Case 3 : After an extended period in intensive care for septicemia and pelvic infection secondary to a surgically-repaired rectal perforation, a 46 year-old man displayed acute tracheal dyspnea due to a sub-glottic stenosis. After 127 laser shots (50 watts, 0.7 second) in a single session, this concentric stenosis located just below the vocal cords was opened from 4 mm to 8.5 mm. The results have been stable for 17 months.

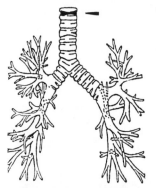 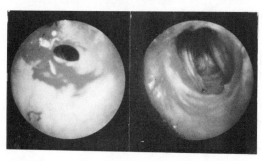

INCIDENTS OR ACCIDENTS

There is a certain amount of risk involved in any good therapeutic technique and laser resection is no exception. Laser accidents can result either from the anesthetic procedure :
- hypoxemia and its cardiac complications : arrhythmia, bradycardia, and cardiac arrest
- adverse reactions to anesthesic drugs especially altesin or from the laser technique itself :
    - hemorrhage during or after resection
    - organ perforation during or after resection
    - post-operative infection
The distinction between anesthesia and technique-related accidents is obviously artificial. Hypoxemia, for example, can be secondary to

hemorrhaging as well as anesthesia. Thus the responsibility of maintaining proper ventilation falls on both the anesthetist and the operator.

INCIDENTS OR ACCIDENTS

ANESTHESIC PROBLEM
local : no cases
general : bradycardias   2 cases (controlled)
          cardiac arrest   2 cases (revived)
          anoxia on awakening   1 case (reversed)
          cardiovascular collapse 2 cases (remedied)

OTHER PROBLEMS
organ perforation   no case
post operative infection   no case
hemorrhaging
- during treatment   11 cases 250 cc
                           (3 cases 700 cc)
- during post operative period (stopped in second session) 1 case

All accidents occurred in patients with malignant tumors except one bradycardia in a case involving a very tight stenosis.

DISCUSSION

Three years of experience with the laser has provided us with a good idea of its utility. By far its most important use is in removing growths obstructing the trachea or bronchial passages. Such treatment is obviously necessary for malignant tumors and, in our opinion, is equally useful for benign tumors of unknown extension outside the bronchus. The repeatability of treatment is attested to by the fact that one adenoid cystic carcinoma was resected 6 times over a 22 month period. Tracheal stenosis can also be submitted to laser treatment as long as it is concentric in form and has no extrinsic complications. For bottle-neck stenosis with extrinsic complications dilatation is mandatory. Follow-up is as yet too brief to allow accurate assessment of long term stability. We only treated patients who were inoperable or had suffered a post-operative recurrence. The Yag laser can also be used to remove granulomas and to section suture threads. It is quite efficient in stopping bronchial hemorrhaging particularly for patients having undergone a tracheotomy in intensive care. The laser can serve to dislodge and remove tissue-embedded foreign bodies with no bleeding. It also appears possible to totally or partially disintegrate soft material such as plastic, wood, or plant. In very stubborn cases, the laser can be used to carve a "handle" on a tissue-embedded foreign body. The choice of anesthesia depends on the indication involved. For large tumors in the trachea or main stem bronchus and for stenosis requiring dilation the open tube is used under general anesthesia. For all other indications a local anesthesia is sufficient. We attribute our low complication and zero fatality rate to the fact that for all high risk patients we make use of an open tube which insures proper ventilation and obviates management of any incident during treatment.

REFERENCES

A 100 page description of our technique and a full bibliography is contained in the "Handbook of Yag Laser Surgery" which may be obtained by writing to our unit.

CHAPTER 9

Nd:YAG LASER APPLICATIONS IN PULMONARY

AND ENDOBRONCHIAL LESIONS

Principal Author:

Michael Unger, M.D., F.C.C.P.
Presbyterian-University of Pennsylvania
  Medical Center
51 North 39th Street
Philadelphia, PA 19104

Nd:YAG LASER APPLICATIONS IN PULMONARY AND ENDOBRONCHIAL LESIONS

UNGER, MICHAEL, M.D., F.C.C.P., ATKINSON, G. WILLIAM, M.D.,F.C.C.P.
Presbyterian-University of Pennsylvania Medical Center, 51 North 39th Street,
Philadelphia, PA 19104

ABSTRACT

Recent developments in Neodymium Yittrium Aluminium Garnet (Nd:YAG)
Lasers and fiberoptic light guide technologies opened up new opportunities
in the therapy of the most frequently occurring carcinoma in man - lung
cancer.

Thorough understanding of basic laser principles and the study of
biological interaction with tissue are necessary prior to technical manipulation.

The data from the clinical study of 30 patients with endobronchial
obstruction are presented. They are further supported by illustrative
examples showing the efficacy of the Nd:YAG Photoresection Therapy. The
results prove that this is a very promising technique in the palliative
therapy of life-threatening endobronchial carcinoma or intractable hemoptysis. It also shows that in a majority of cases the Nd:YAG endobronchial
photoresection and photocoagulation can be performed safely under topical
anesthesia.

INTRODUCTION

Lung cancer is the most frequent carcinoma in man [1]. The histology
of the tumor and its anatomic extent are among the primary factors dictating
the selection of therapeutic approaches. The survival of patients with this
disease is a function of treatment, its availability, its effectiveness and
its applicability. Until now the accepted therapeutic modalities included
surgery, radiation therapy and chemotherapy.

Although introduction of the CO_2 Lasers in the therapeutic armamentarium found also some tracheal applications, it was the possibility of fiberoptic transmission of the Laser beams which opened new approaches in
diagnosis and therapy of endobronchial neoplasms as well as other non-
malignant pathologic manifestations [2]. The two most applicable types of
Lasers were the Argon (Ar) and Neodymium-Yittrium Aluminum Garnet (Nd:YAG)
[3,4].

BIOPHYSICS

Understanding of the basic physical principles of different laser
beams and their biological interactions with the tissue is essential prior
to diagnostic or therapeutic manipulations (TABLE 1) [5]. Each of these
lasers has its potential advantages and disadvantages which have to be
weighed in their utilization. Different tissues have different properties
of absorption (α) and scattering (β) of the laser beams. These characteristics, in major part, are dependent on the specific wave lengths (λ)
of the given laser beams. It is obvious then that as far as the thermal
effects are concerned they will be different with each one of the lasers
[6,7].

© 1983 by Elsevier Science Publishing Co., Inc.
Neodymium-YAG Laser in Medicine and Surgery, Joffe, Muckerheide, and Goldman, editors

TABLE I. Different laser characteristics.

Laser Material	CO_2 gas	Ar gas	Nd:YAG crystal
Wave Length (nm)	10,600	500	1,060
Transmission System	mirrors	fiberoptic	fiberoptic
Absorption in Tissues	high	selective high in blood	low
Coagulation Effects	low	medium	high
Cutting Effect	high	low	low

If cutting or vaporization with a shallow depth of penetration is required, the CO_2 Laser would be the tool of choice [6]. This is due to its very strong absorption in the tissues and its water content on one hand, and minimal scattering on the other. The absorbed electromagnetic energy is transformed into heat energy which can reach high levels necessary for vaporization of the cells.

The Nd:YAG Laser with its infrared wave length has a much lower coefficient of absorption (α), but a much higher coefficient of scattering (β). This will permit increased depth and extent of penetration resulting in a much deeper area of coagulation necrosis. It is, however, important to remember that with the decrease in water content and carbonization, the scattering coefficient diminishes in favor of higher absorption, resulting once more in intense vaporization.

The thermal effects of the Argon Laser are dependent on the blood content of the tissue since this laser has characteristically a very high coefficient of absorption by the red blood cells. Due to Nd:YAG's much lower absorption coefficient in the blood, once more the depth of penetration of this laser beam is increased as long as the blood is not coagulated.

These physical properties of the Nd:YAG Laser, and the biological tissue responses, permit its utilization in endobronchial photocoagulation and photoresection in patients with neoplasms.

METHODOLOGY

All the patients considered for endobronchial laser photoresection therapy (P.R.T.) in our institution had previously-documented neoplasms obstructing major bronchi or the trachea. In most of the cases, these were primary lung tumors, but in some of them the obstruction of the lumen of the airways was due to a metastatic lesion of another origin. As mandated by the Institutional Review Committee, prior to signing a specific consent, the patients received detailed explanations concerning the procedure, its benefits and risks.

All of the patients were to a certain degree in respiratory insufficiency. Some of these, however, presented in severe respiratory failure
due to either primary endobronchial obstruction by a neoplasm judged
unresectable by standard criteria, or to recurrent endobronchial malignancy
and intractable hemoptysis. In one case, surgery was suggested to a thirty-
six year old man with a carcinoid tumor; however, he adamantly refused any
thoracotomy, and opted instead for palliative Nd:YAG Laser photoresection.
The procedures were duly recorded, and endobronchial documentation of
different stages of the P.R.T. on each patient was maintained on videotape.

All of the procedures reported from our institution were performed
utilizing the MediLas 2 Nd:YAG Laser. This equipment is capable of
delivering from 10 watts to 100 watts of power. The effective power,
however, at the tip of the flexible quartz light guide is in the range of
80-90% of the output at the head. The machine is capable of delivering
pulses ranging from 0.1 second with increments of 1/10 of a second up to
9.9 seconds. We found, however, that in endobronchial usage it would be
for the reasons of efficiency or, above all, safety that the pulse length
should not exceed one second. The most useful pulse time ranged between
0.4 to 0.8 seconds.

The machine is also equipped with a low power (2mw) Ne-He laser with
the wave length of 630 nm transmitted through the same light guide fiber.
This strong red light beam permits precise aiming at the target tissue. A
continuous coaxial flow of compressed air around the light guide fiber
assures the cooling of the tip of the fiber as well as dispersion of fumes
and debris. The laser light guide was inserted through the working channel
of a fiberoptic bronchoscope. All of our procedures were done under topical
anesthesia. This, in our opinion, permits useful patient cooperation, and
reduces the risks of general anesthesia as well as the cost of the procedure
[8].

The endobronchial lesions visible through the fiberoptic bronchoscope
are evaluated to determine the insertion point of the base of the tumor
versus the side unattached to the bronchial wall. With the help of the
Ne-He laser beam the invisible therapeutic beam of the Nd:YAG is directed
as much as possible in parallel to the bronchial wall of the partially
obstructed lumen. Occasionally, the aim might be tangential, but never
perpendicular to the wall of the bronchus on which the tumor or obstruction
is located. Utilizing the basic properties of the Nd:YAG Laser, we proceed
with in-depth coagulation in an attempt to reduce the vascular supply to
the tumor, and also possibly reducing its size. This is generally achieved
with energies ranging between 40-50 watts, and pulse time between 0.6
seconds and 0.8 seconds. The visible blanching, drying and shrinking of the
radiated tissue is observed. It is important to notice once more that at
that point the scattering effect in the tissue is increased. The above
energy levels and pulse time setups are also used to stop bleeding. The
total energy applied then is in the range of 150 joules to and around the
bleeding source. After this initial phase, we proceed with vaporization of
the tissue. This is generally achieved with the same or higher energies
(up to 80 watts) and shorter pulses of 0.5 seconds. Vaporization of vascular
tissue requires much higher total energy in the range of 15,000-20,000 joules.
We also noticed that tumors partially necrotized previously or treated
recently with radiotherapy require lower doses of energy to achieve vaporization. With progressive formation of charred tissue, the absorption of

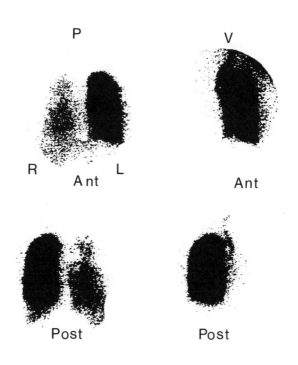

Figure 1. Pre-Laser Scans

We regret that the sequence of pages is incorrect in chapter 9, **"Nd-YAG Laser Applications in
Pulmonary and Endobronchial Lesions."** Please note
that the text on page 79 should immediately follow
the text on page 74 and should precede Figure 1 on
page 75. The remaining sequence is correct.

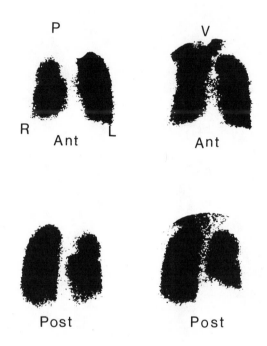

FIG. 2   Post-laser scans

B. Recurrence and Extension of Lung Carcinoma - In a sixty-year old
man, with a previously resected left lower lobe for squamous cell carcinoma,
the tumor recurred and obstructed the left main stem bronchus.   The mass
produced complete atelectasis of the remaining left lung (FIG.3) resulting
in post obstructive pneumonia and sepsis.   In spite of repeated radiation
therapy and antimicrobial therapy, the patient's condition deteriorated
rapidly.   After the first treatment session with the Nd:YAG Laser, patency
of the bronchus was restored permitting drainage of purulent secretions with
rapid clinical improvement and resolution of the life threatening infection.
Additional sessions restored normal ventilation to this area as seen in
(FIG.4).

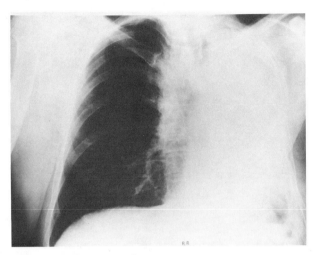

Fig. 3.   Pre-laser chest x-ray.

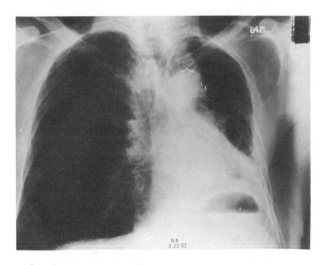

Fig. 4.   Post-laser chest x-ray.

C. Metastatic Carcinoma to the Lung – A fifty-six year old man with previously documented renal cell carcinoma underwent nephrectomy. In spite of radiation therapy and various protocols of chemotherapy he developed multiple lung metastasis. One of them was localized in the left main stem bronchus resulting in hemoptysis, infection and complete atelectasis of the left lung (FIG.5). Successful Nd:YAG Laser endobronchial P.R.T. resulted in reopening of the left main stem bronchus and improved ventilation (FIG.6) and rapid clinical improvement.

78

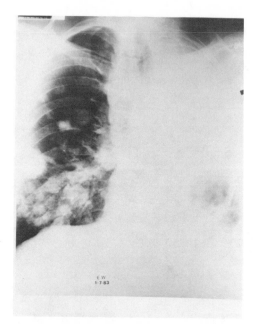

Fig. 5. Pre-laser chest x-ray.

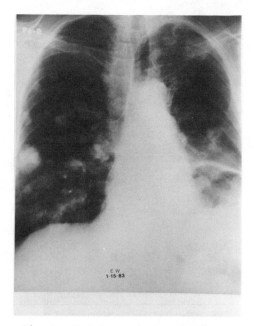

Fig. 6. Post-laser chest x-ray.

the laser beam is markedly increased in this area. This also produces
significant heat and plasma. Laser beam impact in this area may result
then in formation of sparks and combustion of the organic material. Whenever possible, we attempt then to remove the charred surface by mechanical
means using increased suction or biopsy forceps. The most significant
charring occurs in cases of coagulated bleeding.

The immediate results were considered excellent when patency of the
obstructed bronchus and no bleeding was achieved. These results correlated
with clinical and symptomatic improvement. They were classified as fair if
the therapy resulted in only partial patency, but with some improvement of
ventilation and/or symptoms. The results were poor if the hemostasis was
complete, but no patency or ventilation of the obstructed area could be
achieved in spite of removal of the bulk of the tumor. Unsuccessful results
would be considered if the patient's condition deteriorated as a consequence
of the YAG photoradiation therapy.

CLINICAL DATA

We report here data from the ongoing study at Presbyterian-University
of Pennsylvania Medical Center. Thirty symptomatic patients with previously-
documented neoplastic obstruction of the trachea or bronchi underwent sixty-
eight sessions of Nd:YAG Laser P.R.T. Anatomical distribution of these
tumors was as follows: six tumors were located in the trachea, three in the
right and left main stem bronchi (two of them involving the carina), six in
the right main stem, five in the left main stem bronchus. Four tumors
obstructed the right upper lobe, and four involved the left upper lobe. One
was situated in the right bronchus intermedius and one in the right middle
lobe. One neoplastic process blocked the left lower lobe and one the
lingula. From the histologic standpoint, in this group there were eighteen
epidermoid primary lung carcinomas, two adenocarcinomas, two mixed tumors,
one poorly differentiated, one papilloma, one patient presented with
carcinoid tumor, and four patients with metastatic carcinoma from the colon,
kidney, esophagus and larynx respectively. We also successfully treated a
case of foreign body (sutures) granuloma. Various tissue types responded
differently, and not in clearly predictable fashion to the amount of Nd:YAG
Laser energy applied. Three illustrative clinical examples are presented.

A. Primary Lung Carcinoma - (FIG.1) Shows a pretreatment ventilation
(V) and perfusion (P) lung scan with a severely reduced perfusion and absent
ventilation of the right lung in a fifty-seven year old woman. The voluminous squamous cell carcinoma was localized in the junction of the lower
trachea and the right main stem bronchus. Nd:YAG P.R.T. performed in two
sessions restored the patency of the right main stem bronchus and the lower
trachea. Symptomatic improvement was already remarkable after first
treatment. Repeat ventilation and perfusion scan (FIG.2) shows restoration
of ventilation and perfusion to the right lung.

In these three cases, as well as in thirteen others out of the total
of twenty-six cases, the results were excellent. This includes also a
dramatic case of a patient in respiratory failure being mechanically
ventilated due to multiple extensive tracheal tumors (squamous cell
carcinoma) localized between the vocal cords and the carina. Nd:YAG Laser
photoresection permitted vaporization of the bulk of the tumors allowing
extubation and eventual return to normal daily activities. In five cases,
the results were considered fair, thus achieving only partial restoration
of patency. In two of them there was an involvement of the carina. Although
debulking of the tumor mass and good hemostasis was achieved in the remaining five cases, we could not restore their bronchial patency. The results
were then poor.

In our series of patients, no bronchial perforation or death resulted
as a consequence of laser therapy. In one case of treatment of an obstruction of the right upper lobe bronchus, after partial patency was achieved,
open drainage of post obstructive pneumonia produced spillage of pus to the
lower lobe bronchi with formation of a new abscess. This, however, was
successfully treated with antimicrobial therapy. Most of the patients
presented with some degree of hypoxemia when breathing room air, none
suffered any complications as a result of Laser P.R.T., although the
procedure was performed without supplemental O_2 during the lasering period.
Endobronchial combustion, although reported by others, did not occur in
any of our cases [9,10,11]. Neither were we faced with problems of significant bleeding in spite of the hemorrhagic nature of some of the tumors.

We attribute a very low rate of complications in this group to be due
in part to the fact that all of our procedures were done only under topical
anesthesia, allowing full patient cooperation, and reducing the risk of
complications of general anesthesia, intubation and mechanical ventilation.
All the patients tolerated the procedure very well, and only on two occasions
was smoke generated during the vaporization of the tumor a minor irritant
to the patient.

SUMMARY

Rapid expansion of laser development and medical applications of this
new technology require thorough understanding of laser physics and interaction of lasers in living tissue. Because of some of its characteristics,
the Nd:YAG Laser is very suitable for endobronchial applications. Usage
of this laser proves to be a very promising technique in palliative therapy
of life threatening endobronchial carcinoma with airway obstruction or
intractible hemoptysis. It improves the patient's life quality, and their
chances of immediate survival.

The experience proves also that the procedures can be done safely in
most cases through the fiberoptic bronchoscope utilizing only topical
anesthesia, thus reducing the risk of complications to the patient, and
minimizing the cost of the operation. Unfortunately, the power density
or energy density necessary for total vaporization of endobronchial tumors
is variable, and at the present time cannot be accurately predicted.

REFERENCES

1. Ca-A Cancer Journal for Clinicians. Published by the American Cancer Society, 33, No. 1 (1983).

2. E.G. La Foret, R.L. Berger, C.W. Vaughan, Carcinoma obstructing the trachea. Treatment by laser resection. N. Engl. J. Med. 294, 941 (1976).

3. J.C. McDougall, D.E. Cortese, Neodymium YAG Laser Therapy of Malignant Airways Obstruction. Mayo Clin. Proc. 53, 35-39 (1983).

4. J.F. Dumon, E. Reboud, L. Garbe, F. Aucomte, B. Meric, Treatment of Tracheobronchial Lesions by Laser Photoresection. Chest 81, 278-284 (1982).

5. A. Hofstetter, F. Frank, The Neodymium-Yag Laser in Urology. Edit. Roche Switz. (1980).

6. L. Baldassarre, Thermal effects of Nd:YAG and CO_2 lasers on biological tissues. Boll. Soc. Ital. Biol. Sper. 58, 320-326 (1982).

7. G. Godlewski, L. Miro, J.M. Chevalier, J.P. Bureau, Experimental comparative study on morphological effects of different lasers on the liver. Res. Exp. Med. (Berl) 180, 50-57 (1982).

8. G. Vourc'h, M.L. Tannieres, L. Toty, C. Personne, Anaesthetic management of tracheal surgery using the Nd:YAG Laser. Br. J. Anaesth. 52 993-997 (1980).

9. C.A. Hirshman, J. Smith, Indirect ignition of the tracheal tube during CO_2 laser surgery. Arch. Otolaryngol. 106, 639-641 (1980).

10. K.R. Casey, Personal Communication.

11. A.F. Gelb, Personal Communication.

CHAPTER 10

THE Nd:YAG LASER IN UROLOGY

Principal Author:

A. Hofstetter
Department of Urology
Municipal Hospital Thalkirchner Str. 48
D-8000 Munich 2
Germany

84

The Neodymium-YAG Laser in Urology

A. Hofstetter*, F. Frank**, E. Keiditsch***
*Department of Urology, Municipal Hospital Thalkirchner Str.48
 D-8000 Munich 2
** Messerschmitt-Bölkow-Blohm GmbH, D-8012 Ottobrunn
*** Department of Pathology, Municipal Hospital Kölner Platz 1
 D-8000 Munich 40

1. Introduction

The endoscopic application of neodymium-YAG lasers in gastroenterology in
1975 (1) for haemostasis in the stomach and the intestinal tract was
followed directly by the endoscopic application of these lasers in urology
for tumor destroying (2,3). Here too the first experiments were performed
on gas-filled bladders. The fibre systems available for endoscopic transmission of the laser power made it necessary to use rigid endoscopes
with shutoff windows or deflecting prisms   (4). It was particularly
the contamination of these windows and prisms at the distal end of
the laser endoscopes and the problem of reaching as much of the surface
of the bladder wall as possible, that suggested that this approach had no
prospects for routine clinical application. The development of suitable,
mechanically very strong, transmission systems and special laser
urethrocystoscopes (5,6) that could be used in a normally water-filled
bladder, provided the technical prerequisites for applying the neodymium-
YAG laser to the treatment of bladder tumours.

Prior to the application at the clinical level, it was necessary to
establish an optimal dose of the radiation. The neodymium-YAG laser
irradiation results in a deep, conical zone of coagulation necrosis
affecting all layers of the bladder wall down to the serosa, without
causing primary ablation of the tissue. Depending on the dosage, the
coagulation reaches to a depth of 2 to 6 mm, (7) Owing to the fact
that, depending on the consistency of the bladder tissue, 20 to 30%
of the neodymium-YAG laser radiation penetrates the bladder wall as a
result of forward scattering (8,9), there is a risk that neighbouring
organs will be affected, such as adjacent intestinal loops, especially
in the region of the rear wall of the bladder. In addition to the
transmitted radiation, thermal conduction results in some heating
up of the neigbouring organs.

An optimal dose of irradiation is one that completely destroys the
bladder-wall tumours by thermal action, without causing damage to
adjacent organs. The inadequacy of knowledge concerning the thermal
and optical parameters of tissue meant that exact statements on the
production of heat in the tissue, and especially in the bladder, after
neodymium-YAG laser irradiation, and the associated tissue alterations,
could only be based on temperature measurements in the irradiated tissue.

In addition, to optimize the dosage it was necessary to know the exact thickness of the irradiated bladder wall region. To determine the irradiation parameters exactly, the measurement methods must have a high degree of accuracy in the determinations of the bladder-wall thickness and the temperature and they must be applicable in vivo (10,11). For transurethral tissue measurements a special internal ultrasonic transducer has been developed,which is maneuvered into direct contact with the inner wall of the bladder (12,13).

In view of the small wall thicknesses and the small volume of tissue that is heated during the irradiation, initially only a contactless temperature measurement can be considered. Only thus can it be guaranteed that no heat will escape through the measuring instrument and that no direct heating can occur as a result of absorption of the laser radiation, which would falsify the result obtained. The thermocamera is suitable for a contactless measurement of surface temperatures.

A therapeutically optimal dosage was first established in orienting investigations on rabbits, the temperature being measured on various bladder-wall thicknesses.

By performing temperature measurements on fresh human bladder and intestine preparations, it was possible to check on the effect of the dosage established in the preliminary investigations performed on animals.

While carrying out a cystectomy it was possible to perform intraoperative measurements on a living, perfused human bladder, using semiconductor insertion sensors for temperature measurements, calibrated with the thermocamera.

At a power of 45 W maintained for 4 to 5 sec the critical coagulation temperature on the outer bladder wall is not reached by intravesicular irradiation of the human bladder with the neodymium-YAG laser. Subsequent histological examination, made possible by removal of the bladder, revealed depths of necrosis up to 6 mm in the irradiated regions (14,15,16)

A bladder wall tumour extending inwards by up to 5 mm can accordingly be treated satisfactorily with a neodymium-YAG laser power of 45 to 50 W and an exposure time of 2 to 4 sec at the individual irradiation sites. The laser beam should be scanned in lines over the tumour. Adequate protection of adjacent intestinal loops against transmitted radiation is afforded when the bladder wall is of normal thickness.

To the urologist, the basic possiblility of laser coagulation of the tissue without direct contact means that in the external genital region the neodymium-YAG laser can be used for the treatment of condylomata acuminata, carcinomas of the penis and urethra, and of malignant melanomas. In addition to the complete necrotization of the tumour that it brings about, the external use of the laser yields the advantage of a bloodless manner of working (17,18,19).

2. Clinical application

Indications

As already stated, the neodymium-YAG laser can be used to destroy tumour tissue. The specific advantages afforded by the use of the laser are as follows:

- contactless and bloodless obliteration of the tumour, interruption of lymph-drainage (20)
- anaesthesia is unnecessary for endoscopic use; only adapted sedation is required, and thus the treatment can also be extended to outpatient clinics;
- there is no need for post-operative drainage of the bladder by a transurethral catheter, and
- the intervention times are short.

These advantages also determine the indications.

For endoscopic use of the laser, the indications are all tumours that can be eliminated by the neodymium-YAG laser, i.e. tumours up to the size of the ball of the thumb, spreading over an area in carpet-like manner, without metastases(pT_A - pT_2 - N_o - M_o). Moreover, in the case of large and outward-growing tumours, laser coagulation of the tumour bed after removal of the exophytic portion with an electric loop appears to be advantageous.

Further indications for the neodymium-YAG laser are tumours of the external genitals such as carcinomas of the penis and vulva, condylomata acuminata, haemangiomas, and tumours in the urethra, in the ureter (Hofstetter) and in the kidney pelvis.

Irradiation of the tumour bed in residual kidneys after the cutting out of renal adenocarcinomas has proven effective (Hofstetter).

Surgical procedure

The laser system and instruments

For routine clinical use the mediLas YAG coagulation laser made by Messerschmitt-Bölkow-Blohm, Angewandte Technologie GmbH, has proven very successful.

Various laser cysto-urethroscopes are available for the transurethral use of lasers in urology. For outpatients with small bladder tumours of stage TIS and T1 the instrument is composed of a conventional urethro-cystoscope shaft of 19-21 Charr., standard observation optics with variable viewing angles, and a special laser cystoscope attachment. In this arrangement the light guide is passed directly through the ureter-catheter channel of an Albarran instrument. The proximal end of the light guide can be bent through an angle of up to about 80° with the aid of the Albarran lever, so designed that the fibre end is affixed in a protected manner. In addition, the fibre end can be moved in the distal direction to permit exact adjustment of the distance to the irradiation area.

For clinical interventions on larger tumours and for the laser irradiation

of the tumour bed after an electroresection, a 24 Charr. resection
shaft with an oblique tip and a central cock is used instead of the shaft
described above. The greater rinsing effect that can be achieved with
this arrangement permits efficient laser beam irradiation, even when
bleeding occurs. The mobility of the fibre end caused by the angling and
repositioning make it possible to reach and irradiate optimally tumours
at any point on the bladder wall.

For interventions within the urethra in the treatment of urethral carcinomas
and condylomas, use can be made of a modified cystoscope shaft of 15,5
Charr. with an opening at the side of the distal end. In this case there
is no need for the Albarran instrument, since the fibre is passed directly
through the shaft with the observation optics (Frank). Any damage that
could possibly be inflicted on the urethral mucosa by the use of the
Albarran instrument is thus avoided.

For irradiation with the neodymium-YAG laser within the ureter a special
rigid ureteroscope was modified. The instrument with 9-11 french consists
of a kind of telescopic sheath where the viewing optic and the laser-
lightguide is inserted.

For intervention within the kidney pelvis for destroying of urothelial
carcinomas a special flexible pyeloscope was modified.

Endoscopic use of the laser

As in any other transurethral intervention, the patient is placed in
lithotomy position. Anaesthesia is generally unnecessary, appropriate
sedation with diazepam and brevimythal being usally sufficient. To
expand the bladder during the intervention we use sterile physiological
saline. The water-filling also serves to rinse away any bleeding
occurring during the intervention, and thus to prevent local absorption
of the laser beam, which would weaken the coagulating action. The
disadvantages of using water as the rinsing liquid, such as absorption of
the laser radiation in the layer of water between the end of the transmission
system and the bladder wall or the tumour, are negligible when the new
urethrocystoscopes are used and the irradiation distance is reduced.

A whitish coloration of the irradiated tumour tissue indicates that the
treatment is exerting the desired effect. (Fig.1) shows a tumour about
the size of the ball of the thumb before irradiation, (Fig.2) the same
tumour directly after irradiation, and (Fig.3) the local situation
6 weeks later, at which time only a fine scar with in-budding vessels
can still be discerned.

Tumours up to the size of the ball of the thumb are invariably obliterated
in one session with the neodymium-YAG laser. In the case of larger tumours,
on the other hand, the exophytic part is first resected with an electrical
loop deep down into the tunica muscularis. During a second session, 4 to
6 days later, the whole tumour bed and the margins are post-irradiated
with linear scans of the neodymium-YAG laser. Prior to the intervention,
biopsies are taken from the base of the tumour and its edges and from the
immediate surroundings. This process is supplemented by so-called quadrant
biopsy. In the case of smaller tumours, with which a biopsy and primary

removal of the tumour would reduce to one and the same thing, only the neodymium-YAG laser is used. Directly after the irradiation the tumour is removed with the biopsy tweezers and can then be clearly identified and classified histologically.

Since at the most only minor bleeding occurs under the neodymium-YAG laser irradiation, a transurethral catheter is normally unnecessary, a feature that contributes, among other things, to the avoidance of nosocomial infections.

The patient should be supervised for 2 to 3 days after the intervention in order to detect promptly any intestinal perforation, particularly if larger regions on the rear wall of the bladder have been irradiated. With the optimal irradiation dose of up to 45 W established by us, and using water as the rinsing liquid, no such complications have ever been found after the irradiation of almost 1000 tumours to date.

Fig.4,5) Condylomata in the urethra before and after neodymium:YAG laser treatment.
Fig. 6, 7)Ureter tumour before and after laser irradiation and scar formation.

Open applications of laser radiation

This is used whenever the tumour can be reached directly by the laser beam, i.e. primarily for penis carcinomas and condylomata acuminata and also for melanomas and metastases in the external genital region. The irradiation of tumours on the penis is done either after applying a constriction at the root of the penis, or by using a laser handpiece in which a tube is incorporated as a shunt for a jet of gas, so that in the event of major bleeding the emerging blood can be blown away by the gas. Irradiation of the escaping blood, leading to carbonization and wastage of energy, is thus avoided.

A so-called penis block (circumferential subcutaneous injection of 5 to 8 ml of 1% novocaine solution) is first set up at the root of the penis. 3 to 5 min later the tumour is coagulated with the neodymium-YAG laser, taking care to wear special protective goggles to prevent damage to the retina due to reflected laser light.

For condylomata acuminata in the region of the fossa navicularis the fossa is carefully spead out using splitter forceps and the tumor is irradiated. Tumours in the region of the proximal sections of the urethra are treated in the same way as tumours of the bladder, with the aid of an endoscope, and are obliterated by appropriate use of the laser (s.a.), Biopsies are taken before and after the irradiation.

Contraindication

Exclusively endoscopic application of the laser is indicated only for tumours up to the size of the ball of the thumb. Larger tumours should be subjected primarily to transurethral resection with the electric loop. Since only local obliteration of the tumours is possible with the neodymium-YAG laser, the application of laser is ruled out in the case of metastasizing tumours except for the purposes of palliative, local tumour obliteration and haemostasis.

In the case of external use, the laser is only indicated if a radical elimination of the tumour can be envisaged. Advanced stages of penile carcinoma are thus usually directed for surgery, unless only palliative treatment is under consideration.

Clinical results

Since 1st June 1976 we have been using a neodymium-YAG laser at our clinic for endoscopic destruction of bladder tumours and for the treatment of tumours in the external genital region.

Endoscopic use

The efficacy of endoscopic laser therapy used to be limited primarily by the complex transmission systems and by the rigid endoscopes. Now the laser endoscopes with flexible quartz glass fibres which we have had at our disposal since August 1978 allow optimal transurethral use of the neodymium-YAG laser, opening up possibilities of aimed and controllable treatment.

Between August 1978 and August 1980 we treated 132 patients (74 men and 58 women)with bladder tumours. The average age of the patients was 68 years. The tumours were classified in accordance with UICC guidelines. The following treatment groups were thus formed:

1.   Tumours smaller than the ball of the thumb, to be treated solely by the laser.

2.   Transurethral resection in combination with laser coagulation for tumours larger than the ball of the thumb.

        No follow-up treatment with adjuvant chemotherapy was given in these two gropus.

3.   Transurethral resection of the tumour in combination with laser coagulation and adjuvant chemotherapy by instillation of thio-TEPA.

4.   Transurethral resection of the tumour in combination with laser coagulation and instillation of mitomycin C.

The effectiveness of the therapy was evaluated on the basis of the survival rate and the incidence of relapses and was compared with that in a similarly composed group of patients in whom the tumours had been removed exclusively by transurethral electroresection (TUR). Both the laser group and the TUR group included patients requiring so-called palliative therapy, i.e. patients in whom lymph node metastases had already been detected. There were 11 such patients in the laser group and 19 in the TUR group. The remaining patients were assigned to Groups TIS, T_A, T_{1-3}, N_0, and M_0.

Table 1 gives a summary of the tumour classifications in the two groups.

It can be seen that in both groups the tumours were similarly classified
and that the two groups were thus more or less comparable.

Table 2 gives the classification and frequency distribution of the
transitional cell carcinomas, which constituted the main proportion both
in the laser group and in the TUR group. Here too a comparable distribution
was found.

Table 3 gives a synopsis of the lymphogenic metastasization as a function
of the p-stage in both groups.

Patients of these groups come under the heading of palliative therapy,
which was used when the general condition and the advanced age of the
patient no longer permitted radical surgery with lymphadenectomy. These
patients predominated among the mortalities.

Fig.8 shows the survival rates after endoscopic laser irradiation and
after the transurethral electroresection of bladder tumours.

Table 4 shows that in the case of smaller tumours no relapses could
be detected 2 years after the neodymium-YAG laser treatment. It should
be mentioned at this point, however, that the number of cases was
relatively low.

In Table 5 relapse rates between 17 and 40%, depending on the grade of
the primary tumour, are found after 2 years for larger primary tumours
and a larger number of cases. Tables 6 and 7 show a relapse rate between
30 and 50% after 2 years for patients on whom adjuvant chemotherapy was
used, this chemotherapy always involved more than 8 instillations of thio-
TEPA or mitomycin-C.

External use

In the period between January 1977 and September 1981 we treated with
the neodymium-YAG laser 17 patients suffering from carcinomas of the
penis (squamous epithelium carcinomas) in stages T_1 and T_2.
A malignant melanoma of the glans penis was also subjected to neodymium-
YAG laser irradiation.

The patients were aged between 39 and 81; of these 11 were followed up
for between 10 and 39 months. The results are summarized in Table 8. Seven
patients free from metastases did not suffer any local relapse in
the follow-up period up to 30th September 1981, and there was no
metastatic involvement of the regional lymph nodes. In 2 patients with
T_1 and T_2 tumours lymph dissection was carried out for inguinal lymph
nodes in addition to the local therapy. To date, after 11 and 39 months,
both these patients have been free from tumours. One patient in stage
T_2, N_3, M_1 underwent lymphadenectomy and chemotherapy in addition to
the local treatment. A relapse the size of a grain of rice was found on
the glans penis. This patient died of metastases 30 months after the start
of the treatment. The patient with primary melanoma of the glans and
inguinal lymph node metastases died of the disease 20 months after the
start of the therapy. The penis itself was confirmed by biopsy to be
free from tumours.

Among the more than 30 patients with condylomata acuminata we observed only 2 cases of relapse, which were apparently due to deficient primary irradiation.

Histological examination immediately after the laser irradiation clearly confirmed thorough denaturation of the irradiated tissue.

In addition to condylomata acuminata we used the neodymium-YAG laser for the treatment of urethral carcinomas, urethral caruncles, and carcinomas and condylomata acuminata of the vulva.

3.   Critical appraisal of the use of lasers in urology

Our experience to date with the endoscopic application of the laser demonstrates the superiority of this technique as regards radicality but also in respect of the operative procedure. This seems to be shown by a controlled, prospective study during the last two years. Nevertheless, a definitive evaluation is still impossible. On the other hand, our experience with the external use of the laser has been convincing. Only the high cost and the lack of experience remain as obstacles to a wider use of the neodymium-YAG laser in medicine.

Table 1   Classification of Urinary Bladder Tumours in 132 Patients of

the Laser Group (74m/58w) and In 235 Patients in a TUR-Group

(192m/43w)

	Laser Group (%)	TUR-Group (%)
Papilloma	6.0	4.0
Carcinoma in situ	1.5	2.0
Transitional cell carcinoma	87.0	89.5
Rare tumours	5.0	3.0
Metastases of extravesical primary tumours	0.5	1.5
	100.0	100.0

Table 2   Classification and Incidence Distribution of Transitional

Cell Carcinoma in % Out of Table 1

G ＼ T	Laser Group				TUR-Group			
	1	2	3	Undifferentiated Carcinoma	1	2	3	Undifferentiated Carcinoma
a	26.0	11.0	1.5	--	25.0	5.0	1.0	--
1	9.0	9.0	2.0	1.0	11.0	11.0	3.0	1.5
2	--	2.0	8.5	0.5	4.0	7.0	5.0	0.5
3	--	2.0	10.0	--	--	3.0	8.0	0.5
4	--	--	4.5	--	--	--	4.0	--
	35.0	24.0	26.5	1.5	40.0	26.0	21.0	2.5

Table 3   Lymphogenous Formation of Metastases Dependent

on the T-Stage

	Laser Group N_{1-3} (%)	TUR Group N_{1-3} (%)
T_1	3.5	4.5
T_2	20.0	22.0
T_3	25.0	28.5
T_4	100.0	100.0

Table 4   Recurrence of Tumour after Laser-Coagulation

Dependent on Grading

Therapeutic Method		Number of Patients	Relapses after 2 years (n) (%)	
Nd:YAG Laser Coagulation	G_0	5	-	-
(tumour's diameter <1.5 cm)	G_1	2	-	-
	G_2	1	-	-
	G_3	-	-	-

Table 5   Recurrence of Tumor after Laser-Coagulation

Dependent of Grading

Therapeutic Method		Number of Patients	Relapses after 2 years	
			(n)	(%)
TUR and Laser coagulation (tumor's diameter >1.5 cm)	G_0	5	–	–
	G_1	18	3	17
	G_2	8	3	37
	G_3	5	2	40

Table 6   Recurrence of a Tumor after Laser-Coagulation

Dependent on Grading

Therapeutic Method		Number of Patients	Relapses after 2 years	
			(n)	(%)
TUR and Laser coagulation and Thiotepa	G_0	1	1	–
	G_1	14	7	50
	G_2	1	–	–
	G_3	–	–	–

Table 7   Recurrence of a Tumour after Laser-Coagulation
Dependent on Grading

Therapeutic Method		Number of Patients	Relapses after 2 years (n)	(%)
TUR and laser-coagulation and Mitomycin C	G_0	-	-	-
	G_1	3	1	33
	G_2	23	7	30
	G_3	13	5	38

Tumor Classification TREATMENT	Number of patients	Age (years)	Follow-up up to 9-30-81 (months)	Local Relapse	Palpable Lymphnodes
Laserirradiation					
$T_1\ N_0\ M_0$	6	39-77	10-27	0	0
$T_2\ N_0\ M_0$	1	63	24	0	0
Laser + Lymphadenectomy					
$T_1\ N_2\ M_0$	1	48	39	0	0
$T_2\ N_2\ M_0$	1	54	11	0	0
Laser + Lymphadenectomy + Chemotherapy					
$T_2\ N_3\ M_1$	1	59	30 †	1	fixed nodes
$T_2\ N_2\ M_0$(Melanoma)	1	61	24 †	0	0

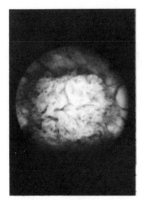

Fig.1: Bladder tumour before
laser irradiation

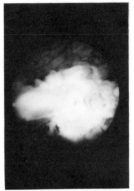

Fig.2: Tumour directly after
irradiation

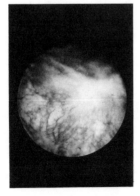

Fig.3: Local situation
6 weeks after laser
irradiation

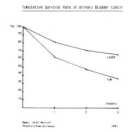

Cumulative Survival Rate in Urinary Bladder Cancer

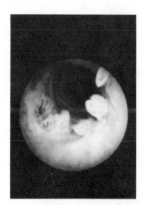

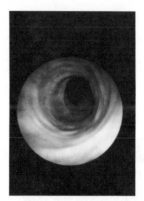

Fig.4: Condylomata in the
urethra before Nd:YAG
laser irradiation

Fig.5: 8 weeks after irradiation
of condylomata in the urethra

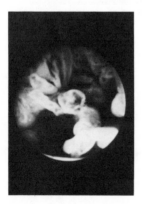

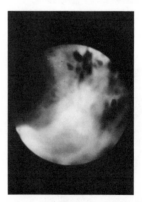

Fig.6: Uretertumours

Fig.7: 6 weeks after Nd:YAG laser
irradiation of ureter-
tumours

1.) KIEFERHABER, P., NATH, G, MORITZ, K.:
   Endoscopical Control of massive Gastrointestinal Hemorrhage by
   Irradiation with a High-Power Neodym-YAG-Laser
   Progr. Surg. 15, 140, 1977

2.) HOFSTETTER,A., STAEHLER,G., KEIDITSCH,E.
   Experimentelle Erzeugung von malignen Tumoren an der Kaninchenharn-
   blase; Fortschr.Med. 95, 346, 1977

3.) STAEHLER,G., HOFSTETTER,A., SCHMIEDT,E., KEIDITSCH,E., ROTHER, W.,
   GORISCH,W., WEINBERG,W.:
   Endoskopische Laser-Bestrahlung von Blasentumoren des Menschen;
   Fortschr.Med. 95, 1, 1977

4.) STAEHLER,G., HOFSTETTER,A., FRANK,F., HALLDORSSON,Th.:
   Ein Zystoskop für die Applikation von Neodym-YAG-Laserstrahlen zur
   Zerstörung von Blasentumoren;
   akt.uro. 9, 271, 1978

5.) HOFSTETTER,A., FRANK, F.:
   Ein neues Laser-Endoskop zur Bestrahlung von Blasentumoren;
   Fortschr.Med. 97, 232, 1979

6.) FRANK,F., HOFSTETTER,A., BÖWERING,R., KEIDITSCH,E.:
   Endoscopic application of the Neodymium-YAG-laser in urology,
   biophysical fundamentals and instrumentation;
   Proc.SPIE 211, 36, 1979

7.) HOFSTETTER,A., FRANK, F., et al:
   The Neodymium-YAG laser in urology;
   Basel Editiones Roche, 1980

8.) HALLDORSSON,Th., LANGERHOLC,J.:
   Thermodynamic Analysis of Laser Irradiation of Biological Tissue;
   Appl.Optics 17, 3948, 1978

9.) STAEHLER, G., HALLDORSSON, Th., LANGERHOLC, J., BILGRAM, R.:
   Dosimetry for Neodymium-YAG laser Applications in Urology;
   Lasers Surg. and Med. 1, 191, 1980

10.) PENSEL,J., HOFSTETTER,A., KEIDITSCH,E., ROTHENBERGER,K.,STAEHLER,G,
    FRANK,F., GORISCH,W.:
    Temperature Profile in Space and Time on the Bladder Wall Serosa
    and Time on the Bladder Wall Serosa During Intravesical Laser
    Irradiation;
    in: Laser Surgery III, Part 2, Tel Aviv, 1979

11.) PENSEL,J., HOFSTETTER,A., KEIDITSCH,E., FRANK,F., ROTHENBERGER,K.:
    Tierexperimentelle Untersuchungen zur Frage der Temperaturprofile
    an der Blasenwandserosa bei intravesikaler Neodym-YAG-Laserbe-
    strahlung;
    Abstr.Exp. Urolog. 38, Gräfelfing Demeter, 1980

98

12.) PENSEL,J., ROTHENBERGER,K., HOFSTETTER,A., FRANK,F.:
A-Bild-Sonographie zur Messung der Harnblasenwandstärke;
Fortschr.Med. 98, 1066, 1980

13.) ROTHENBERGER,K., PENSEL,J., HOFSTETTER,A., KEIDITSCH,E., FRANK,F.:
Determination of Invasion of Urinary-Bladder Tumors Using of a new
Transurethral Ultrasonic Method;
NUA 1, 217, 1981

14.) PENSEL,J., HOFSTETTER,A., FRANK,F., KEIDISCH,E., ROTHENBERGER,K.:
Temporal and Spatial Temperature Profile of the Bladder Serosa in
Intravesical Neodymium-YAG laser Irradiation;
Eur.Urol. 7, 298, 1981

15.) ROTHENBERGER,K., PENSEL,J., FRANK,F., KEIDITSCH,E., HOFSTETTER,A.:
Experiments of optimize the dose for endovesical irradiation with
the Neodymium-YAG laser. Investigations in bladders of rats,
rabbits and corpses;
urol.res. 8, 227, 1980

16.) HOFSTETTER,A., FRANK,F., KEIDITSCH,E., BÖWERING,R.:
Endoscopic Neodymium-YAG Laser Application for Destroying Bladder
Tumors;
Eur.Urol. 7, 278, 1981

17.) HOFSTETTER,A., STAEHLER,G., KEIDITSCH,E., FRANK,F.:
Lokale Laser-Bestrahlung eines Peniskarzinoms,
Fortschr.Med. 96, 269, 1978

18.) ROTHENBERGER,K, HOFSTETTER,A., GEIGER,M., BÖWERING,R., FRANK,F.:
Erfahrungsbericht über die externe Anwendung eines Neodym-YAG-
Lasers, Verhandlb. Deutsche Ges.Urolog. 31.Tag.: 241, Berlin,
Heidelberg, New York, Springer-Verlag, 1980

19.) STAEHLER,G.:
Die externe Applikation von Neodym-YAG-Laserstrahlen in der Urologie;
Urologe A 20, 323, 1981

20.) KEIDITSCH,E., STERN,J., ZIMMERMANN,J., HOFSTETTER,A., FRANK,F.,
PENSEL,J., ROTHENBERGER,K.:
Interruption of Urinary Bladder wall lymph drainage by Neodymium-
YAG laser Irradiation;
Transact.LASER Tokyo 1981, 10-48, 1981

CHAPTER 11

TRANSURETHRAL YAG LASER TREATMENT OF BLADDER TUMORS -

RATIONALE, INSTRUMENTATION AND TECHNIQUE

S. Bjorn Lundquist, M.D.
Department of Urology
University Hospital
S-221 85 Lund, Sweden

TRANSURETHRAL YAG LASER TREATMENT OF BLADDER TUMORS - RATIONALE,
INSTRUMENTATION AND TECHNIQUE

S. BJÖRN LUNDQUIST, M.D.
Department of Urology
University Hospital
S-221 85 Lund, Sweden

INTRODUCTION

The general principles for management of bladder carcinoma and histological grading and staging have developed alongside. Proper classification of
a tumor still requires ample biopsy material obtained by TUR. The decision-
making process involves clinician, pathologist, oncologist and patient. The
choice of therapy varies strongly internationally. This is especially marked
in tumors considered to be manageable by the transurethral route alone,
particularly regarding the use of intravesical chemotherapy.

Historical views of tecnniques for transurethral surgical bladder tumor
management

Before 1910, smaller bladder tumors were mechanically snared and removed
along with the cystoscope. Operation under visual control had been available
for only about 20 years at that time. In 1907 surgical diathermy was reported. Already in 1910, the American urologist Erwin Beer reported success
with this technique for coagulation of small bladder tumors. With the simultaneous development of diathermy and transurethral surgery, removal of tumors
by resection was not possible until 1930. Although technology for diathermy
has changed, and the resectoscopes have been improved, the method prevails
as a diagnostic and therapeutic procedure.

The first laser was constructed in 1960, and it was soon realized that
this type of energy could be used in surgery. The past 8 years have seen the
development of Nd:YAG laser for transurethral surgery "under water". The
wavelength is transmitted fairly well through water, and penetrates deep into
biological tissue. Furthermore, it is easily transmitted through flexible
optic fibres at high powers, making it the ideal laser for endoscopic use.
Work with the YAG laser in a rather thin-walled body cavity, such as the urinary bladder, raised many questions calling for an answer before clinical use
could be considered. Thanks to the theoretical and experimental works performed at the MBB Company in collaboration with the clinicians G. Staehler
and A. Hofstetter of Munich (1, 2) the technique could be taken into clinical use. There also exists a vast clinical experience in Western Germany to
date. The experience outside this country is still limited.

Mechanisms of interaction between YAG radiation and biological tissue (regarding transurethral use)

When optical (e.g. laser) energy is absorbed in tissue, heating is effected by conversion to thermal energy. The temperature elevation in a tissue
volume is mainly determined by the amount of energy deposited in it. The
heating velocity depends on the power density (power per unit volume). When
YAG radiation exits from the tip of a fiber under water, some power is lost
by absorption in the water. There is also a certain loss within the fiber itself. Already the heating of water causes a certain scattering.

The power impinging on the tissue surface, thus will be highly dependent
on the length of water path between fibertip and tissue. The residual power
impinging on the tissue surface is partly back-scattered into the water,
partly forward-scattered into the tissue, and partly transmitted. As the
radiation passes through the tissue, scattering phenomena occur and reoccur,
causing a fairly even distribution of power density within a limited volume
of tissue. As the tissue temperature approaches 60°C, which is enough for

necrosis, back-scattering increases, and the in depth heating is limited. Only thermal diffusion will be responsible for deeper heating. This pheno- menon is responsible for significant temperature elevations only at depths of more than some additional tenths of a mm. This excursion in physics (3) is intended to demonstrate that a proper matching of power and timing re- sults in a reproducible coagulation depth.

Present clinical experience of the YAG laser for transurethral coagulation of bladder tumors

The presented German papers deal mainly with experimentally determined safety limits. One clinical report (4) of about 250 patients is not quite conclusive, since the patients were treated with two different laser systems and/or TUR, and after that divided into two separate groups receiving diffe- rent regimes of intravesical chemotherapy. However, it indicates that TUR and laser coagulation are comparable in therapeutical efficacy. Only in one case, where a mistake in excessive energy dose was used, bowel complica- tions occurred. Otherwise, no complications were reported. Even with the now considerably larger material, no complications have been encountered.

WHAT KIND OF TUMORS ARE SUITABLE FOR LASER THERAPY?

Bladder carcinoma is rarely located to one area of the urothelium. Either a large area or multiple small ones have the potential of growing tumors (5, 6). This is the main obstacle in comparing the efficacy of YAG vs TUR (unless you believe in implantation metastases occurring during TUR, since those are abolished with laser therapy).

In my opinion a newly discovered bladder tumor should be graded and staged by TUR. The next few (2-3) new tumors ought to be dealt with in the same way. Once you have established the behaviour of the neoplastic disease you could consider laser therapy. Since there is little doubt that the most usual origin of "new" tumor growth is the urothelium adjacent to the primary tumor, you can consider different methods of destroying this area. A super- ficially extended TUR or diathermy coagulation may be as effective as laser irradiation, but gives you no possibility to determine the depth of damage produced. By laser irradiation you can match power and timing to produce damage only to the mucosal layer.

Tumor grades and stages

G1, pTa - T1 tumors can definitely be treated by laser coagulation if their size does not exceed 10 mm in diameter. G2, pTa - T1 tumors are also suitable, but could be more prone to convert into higher malignancy grades. Thus, if laser therapy is attempted, it should be accompanied by biopsy or at least aspiration cytology. Cytology from voided urine or bladder washings may be insufficient and non-specific to demonstrate conversion into a G3 tumor (7).

In G3, pT1, therapeutical traditions differ. If you have a conservative attitude, TUR can be supplemented by laser in depth coagulation over a large area. The efficacy of this supplementary therapy has to be established by controlled trials.

In poor risk patients with G3, pT2 tumors it is likely that laser coa- gulation can improve results. This also requires controlled trials to be proven.

Certain problems exist in the two G3 groups, since patients have to be matched regarding several different parameters. Multicenter trials have to be designed to give results within a reasonable period of time.

The G1 - G2 patients usually are in stages pTa - T1. Many respond well to intravesical chemotherapy, which means that you may be facing an ethical problem.

Obviously this is an item that has to be discussed between urologists from different countries and of different opinions of the best way to treat different grades and stages of bladder tumors.

INSTRUMENTATION

Basically, the system consists of the laser machine, an optical fiber delivery system and a specially designed Albarran lever insert. Any YAG laser suitable for transurethral use requires a high power, three-phase, main supply. Water supply for cooling and a drainage is also needed.

The laser

There is definitely more urological experience with the MediLas (MBB Company, Munich). I have been using a Fiberlase 100 (Barr & Stroud, Ltd, Glasgow) for more than one year, and in the past few months also the Medi-Las. The Fiberlase has physical dimensions exceeding those of the MediLas, but is still more convenient to move around the OR floor. As the endoscopy room is rather dark during surgery, you will find the LCD read-out of the MediLas difficult to see, while the Fiberlase has large, bright LED displays. If you want to change from the urological fiber system to e.g. a hand held tool, you will need a gas supply. With the Fiberlase you can have the gas connected all the time, and it will be immediately available when needed. With the MediLas, you will have to change the footswitch and connect the gas supply to both footswitch and delivery system. Both lasers have sterilizable adapters for power calibration of the fiber before use.

The delivery system

As when using a diathermy electrode, you need freedom to move the laser fiber tip. The MediLas system is spring-loaded for this purpose, but there is no brake included to lock the fiber in its proper position. Once you get used to it, the problem is small. The Fiberlase system is presently being equipped with a fiber brake, and a system allowing easy positioning of the fiber, at the same time locking it into place. Cleaning, sterilization and desinfection of the systems is another important question. The MediLas system can at present only be desinfected by immersing the distal end in glutaraldehyde solution, or gas sterilized. The Fiberlase system can be fully immersed in glutaraldehyde, autoclaved at $120^{\circ}C$ or gas sterilized.
When you start working with a YAG laser you will no doubt have some damaged fiber tips. This can occur by mechanical force. More usual is that you fire the laser while the tip is in tissue contact. The MediLas fibers have a length of 10-15 mm (3 mm loss with one repair) available for repairs.
The Fiberlase system can be repaired up to 20 times. At this time, the MediLas system has to be replaced, while the Fiberlase system allows for at least a hundred more repairs. The tips are easily repaired by yourself or the technicians of your hospital.

The endoscopic equipment

The conventional Albarran lever is modified to a somewhat larger metal plate of 3-4 mm thickness, and 5 mm length, containing a 1 mm channel for protection and exact guiding of the fiber. To date, these are made only by the Storz Company and the Wolf Company, both German. The Storz one only deflects to about 60°, which makes work in the bladder neck region difficult. The Wolf one deflects to almost 90°, which makes it far more useful. The latter one is used with a standard 19.5 F cystoscope sheath. It is favourable to have 25°, 70° and 110° working telescopes. Wolf also makes a special aspiration cytology catheter, which is useful for obtaining directed specimens. A conventional cross-cut ureteral catheter can also be used. To reach

tumors in the vicinity of the bladder neck I use a retrograde electrode guide for directing the laser fiber. It can also be used with the aspiration
catheter or a flexible biopsy forceps (also supplied by the Wolf Company).
For the routine cystoscopies I prefer the 70° wide angle examining telescope
made by the Wolf Company.

The operating telescopes have to be fitted with protective eye filters,
either permanently, or as a clip-on system.

TECHNIQUE

Safety

It is important to realize that this new technique takes quite some
training. First, you should get acquainted with the laser, the delivery
system and the endoscopic equipment without patients present. All present
personnel should be wearing special protective goggles, even if there is
little risk of dangerous amounts of radiation escaping into the room. If the
OR has windows, these should be provided with blinds. The doors of the OR are
easily interlocked with the laser, so that it cannot be fired without having
all doors shut. Warning lamps and signs outside the room are a must. Training
of OR staff routines is preferrably done, while you find out what the action
of the laser is like on a piece of raw meat. Remember instructions also to
anesthesiologists. It is a good idea to place a pair of goggles outside the
OR door for use in emergencies.

Surgery

Patient information is extremely important, since the word "Laser" takes
most peoples' minds to the horrible beam that was supposed to slice up a
certain secret agent (known as 007) in a movie. As a premedication we use
a somewhat heavier combination than that used before general anesthesia.
Careful anesthesia of the urethra is applied by 2 % Lidocaine®jelly (Astra,
Sweden), 5-10 g, twice with a 10 minute interval.

Following routine cystoscopy and location of tumors, the laser fiber is
introduced all the way into the Albarran lever channel, with the insert held
in your hand. The fiber is calibrated and the laser set to deliver 40-45 W.
The machine is not activated for lasing until you have placed the insert and
are ready for lasing. Check that all OR staff is wearing their goggles (don't
forget the patient). Preset pulse duration to 2-3 seconds. Make sure that
you see the very tip of the laser fiber in the margin of the visual field,
and that you have a good aiming spot (NEVER use a fiber that does not give a
proper aiming beam!). Activate the laser, and you are ready to start. Adjust
the distance between tissue and fiber tip to 1.5-3 mm. When you press the
footswitch, you will see the tissue shrinking and blanching at the end of each
pulse. Work your way around the tumor, and pay special attention to the tumor
base. If you happen to fire a second time at an already coagulated area, you
will have a small evaporization. This is harmless, but should be avoided. If
the distal aspect of the tumor is difficult to reach with the beam, you can
"peel off" some of the coagulated tumor by gentle manipulation (not with
fiber tip!). You are less likely to have this problem with the Wolf equipment
- just change the telescope. After I have finished treating the tumor, I usually increase the power to 60 W, and decrease the pulse duration to 0.5 seconds, and coagulate the 5-10 mm mucosal border surrounding the tumor.

Most patients do not experience any pain, though there may be a few who
do. You can use any irrigating solution, but try to keep the bladder volume
below some 250 ml. If the patient is a "potential prostatic" I give him an
indwelling catheter for a few hours after the operation. It is wise to keep
patients in the hospital for 12-24 hours before you are completely familiar
with the technique.

SUMMARY

The medical care system of Sweden (99 % socialized) would make a YAG laser pay for itself within 2 years, even if used only in urology. With the internationally differing traditions of therapy and medical care systems, the question is not that simple. It is neither quite certain that the medical benefits of the YAG laser in urology alone justify its use. There are however several important applications for the YAG laser in other disciplines. This should be considered, and multidisciplinary use of the machine coordinated at a very early stage, when planning to bring a YAG laser into your hospital permanently.

REFERENCES

1. A. Hofstetter, F. Frank. The Neodynium-YAG Laser in Urology. Roche Scientific Service, Basel. (1980).
2. J. Pensel et al. Temporal and Spatial Temperature Profile of the Bladder Serosa in Intravesical Nd-YAG Laser Irradiation. Eur. Urol. 7, 298-303 (1981).
3. G. Staehler, Th. Halldorsson, J. Langerholc and R. Bilgram. Endoscopic applications of the Nd:YAG Laser in Urology; Theory, Results, Dosimetry. Urol. Res. 9, 45-51 (1981).
4. A. Hofstetter, F. Frank, E. Keiditsch and R. Böwering. Endoscopic Neodymium-YAG Laser Application for Destroying Bladder Tumors. Eur. Urol. 7, 278-282 (1981).
5. H.R. England, A.M.I. Paris and J.P. Blandy. The Correlation of T1 Bladder Tumour History with Prognosis and Follow-up Requirements. Br. J. Urol. 53, 593-597 (1981).
6. Clinical Bladder Cancer. L. Denis, P.H. Smith and M. Pavone-Macaluso, eds. (Plenum Press, New York 1982).
7. T. Farsund. Selective Sampling of Cells for Morphological and Quantitative Cytology of Bladder Epithelium. J. Urol. 128, 267-271 (1982).

CHAPTER 12

Nd:YAG LASER IN UROLOGY

Eric J. Sacknoff, M.D.
Harvard Medical School
Boston, Massachusetts

NEODYMIUM-YAG LASER IN UROLOGY

Eric J. Sacknoff, M.D., F.A.C.S., Harvard Medical Schooo
Instructor in Surgery (Urology), Boston, Massachusetts

INTRODUCTION

The field of urology has enjoyed a rich tradition in endoscopic surgery with the advent of transurethral electrocautery
for bladder and prostate neoplasms. As surgeons collaborated
to improve upon better techniques of tissue removal and destruction, the development of the laser provided yet another
tool for this purpose. It seems only fitting that urologists
would lead the crusade for endoscopic laser surgery; however,
this has not been the case for several reasons. First,
electrocautery has served urology so well that no great need
seemed urgently necessary. Second, the particular physical
properties of the Ruby and CO_2 lasers made endoscopic delivery
either bulky, awkward or technically impossible. Finally,
the research and development costs far outweighed the apparent
benefit over electrocautery. Nevertheless, scientists,
surgeons, and innovators persevered in the field of Neodymium-
YAG (Nd-YAG) laser technology to provide the initial breakthrough for endoscopic urologic laser treatment.

Although the Nd-YAG laser may be used for open surgery
with a hand laser scalpel, this discussion will emphasize
the endoscopic urologic experience. The unique Nd-YAG properties of enhanced power density, low absorption in tissue
and transmission through a flexible fiber provide a versatile
set of functions when adapted to conventional urologic instrumentation. The low power of the Argon laser and the lack of a
fiber delivery system for the CO_2 laser represent significant
limitations for urologic surgery.

HISTORY

After Parsans et al in 1966 first demonstrated that a
laser beam could be used in vivo in the canine bladder under
simulated cystoscopic conditions[1], it became clear that a
delivery system for cystoscopic application was necessary to
transmit the laser energy from the light source to the tissue[2].
In 1970 Mussiggang presented a theoretical description of a
flexible delivery system at the annual meeting of the German
Urological Association[3]. In 1973 Nash developed a flexible
quartz laser waveguide capable of transmitting high power
Nd-YAG and Argon laser light[4]. This early technological breakthrough for delivering Nd-YAG and Argon laser light for operative gastroscopy paved the way for future adaptations in
urology. In 1976 and 1977 Rothauge and Staehler developed
special laser cystoscopes for bladder tumor irradiation[5,6].
For the first time cystoscopic Nd-YAG and Argon laser irradiation of the bladder wall using a flexible quartz fiber light
guide was studied morphologically and histologically[7]. Staehler
et al found that experimental Argon laser irradiation of the
bladder showed good tissue removal without the danger of
perforation. However, bleeding from vessels greater than 1mm
in diameter could not be stopped even though a higher power
density was used [7].

The shallow depth of thermal action of the Argon laser in
bladder tissue influenced other investigators to favor the use

© 1983 by Elsevier Science Publishing Co., Inc.
Neodymium-YAG Laser in Medicine and Surgery, Joffe, Muckerheide, and Goldman, editors

of the Nd-YAG laser in urology. The Nd-YAG laser with its wavelength of 1.06 microns emits a continuous invisible beam in the near infrared region of the electromagnetic spectrum. The absorption in tissue at this wavelength is very slight; while the scattering in the tissue at this wavelength is considerable. This property promotes a uniform distribution of radiation in the tissue to achieve hemostasis and a greater depth of coagulative necrosis[8]. Following the early urologic experience in Germany with the Nd-YAG laser by such pioneers as Staehler, Hofstetter, Frank, and Bulow in the late 1970's, Okada and associates[9] from Japan, Lundquist and associates from Sweden[10], and McPhee and associates from Canada[11], provided further contributions in the early 1980's regarding indications, treatment, technique, and instrument technology in endoscopic bladder tumor surgery.

INSTRUMENTATION

The Nd-YAG laser may be delivered through a flexible light guide made of a quartz glass fiber. Transmission of the beam occurs by successive total internal reflections of light from the laser head of the mobile console through the fiber conductor. The preferred type of quartz fiber used in urology has a diameter of 0.6 mm and is covered with a Teflon sleeve. This strong fiber has an outlet divergence of 10 degrees and a transmission of 85%. The higher outlet beam divergence coupled with a narrow fiber of high mechanical strength allows for simple incorporation into conventional cystoscopes to irradiate larger cross-sectional areas[8]. Since the Nd-YAG laser beam is invisible, a coaxial Helium-Neon pilot beam emits a visible red or green spot on the surgical target site.

Two types of light conductor systems exist: the endoscopic light conductor and the standard light conductor. The endoscopic system has a thinner portion of the fiber unprotected by an outer, flexible metal and plastic tube enabling it to be directly passed into the cystoscope. The standard light conductor is protected along its entire length by a flexible metal and plastic tube so that the outlet end can be adapted to a hand-held focusing device for open surgical use[8].

Early laser cystoscopes adapted for Nd-YAG use were closed off at the outlet end by a window or prism so the light conductor would be protected on all sides. Since these sealed systems became soiled with the heat of tissue char and smoke, it was necessary to clean and cool the sealed window with either gas or water through run off tubes.

The rigid laser cystoscope system as described by Bulow et al consisted of a double tube in which the inner tube contained the light cable and optical system. This inner tube is closed at the distal end by a quartz window. The beam may be focused to a spot 1.5 mm in diameter about 20 mm from the tip of the instrument. Gas, such as carbon dioxide, is introduced between the outer and inner tube with sufficient intensity to cleanse the quartz windows from contaminations by urine, blood, or tissue. The gas also served to dissipate heat absorbed within the system that could destroy the window and potentially the light fiber[12].

The use of the flexible, quartz fiber through a cystoscope with a modified Albarren bridge provides a lever for fiber deflection of almost 90° in a water-filled bladder. No special cleaning or cooling of the light conductor is necessary. This laser cystoscope is superior to the sealed rigid systems because of its high flexibility, low maintenance problems, and its ability to be easily sterilized[8].

McPhee et al believed that the Nd-YAG laser alone offered little therapeutic advantage over conventional transurethral electrocautery unless safe destruction of bladder wall both behind and adjacent to the lesion was achieved. Accordingly, this group modified an ACMI Iglesias resectoscope to accept a 2 mm fiberoptic transmission cable through the center of the cautery loop. The laser probe was arranged at a measured distance of 1 cm from the cautery loop. The tip of the probe was modified to a convex lens to enlarge the spot size from 2.8 mm to 1 cm by increasing the divergant angle from 8 degrees to 36 degrees. The critical probe to mucosa 1 cm distance allowed doses up to 540 joules to be delivered without bladder or bowel perforation[11]. This ingenious instrument which blends both electrocautery and laser technology provides biopsy material to be obtained at the time of treatment and staging.

THERMAL BEHAVIOR ON UROLOGIC TISSUE

To understand the thermal behavior of the Nd-YAG laser on biologic tissue one must have a clear notion of the physical properties of this laser in comparison to the Argon and CO_2 lasers. Since the Nd-YAG is a solid state laser emitting a continuous beam in the near infrared region of the electromagnetic spectrum at a wavelength of 1.06 microns; its transmission through water is high and the absorption within the tissue is slight. Since tissue absorption is slight, the ability of the Nd-YAG laser to scatter both forward and backward through bladder tissue is important. With bladder tissue 2 mm thick in vitro experiments show that the forward scattered power of Nd-YAG laser light through the tissue amounts to only 25-30% of the incident beam; while, the back scattering amounts to 30-40% of the total incoming power. Limitation of applied laser power and irradiation time prevents irreversible thermal damage from forward scattering of radiation to either the target organ (bladder) or adjacent organs (intestines). Furthermore, back scattering through the endoscope may be another potential hazard to the eyes of the surgeon. However, with the appropriate applied dosage to the bladder tissue both the transmitted and back-scattered radiation are emitted in a diffuse form. At controlled power and irradiation time settings this diffuse scattering offers additional protection since the resultant power density to the adjacent perivesical organs is so low[8]. The resultant radiation from the penetrating YAG laser beam produces a deep, homogeneous form of heating scattered over a large volume of tissue rather than to a precise focal spot. The broad coagulative necrosis produced by the Nd-YAG laser is, therefore, distinguished from the more shallow precise crater obtained with the CO_2 or Argon lasers.

At 37-60° C tissue is merely warmed. At 60-65° C proteins are denatured and necrosis occurs. Coagulation necrosis occurring at about 60° C alters the optical tissue properties so that more of the radiation is back scattered and less is

absorbed. The bladder mucosa turns grayish white with limitation of the immediate maximum heating depth. With continued
irradiation, the temperature rises slowly until the tissue
water has been evaporated. Drying occurs at 90-100° C.
Carbonization of the tissue occurring at a few hundred degrees
centrigrade causes increased absorption and decreased back-
scattering of the laser due to the darkening of the tissue.
This tissue darkening seems to be specific to the blood within
the tissue. Obviously, this dangerously high absorption at
high temperatures above coagulation (60°C) imposes specific
limits on penetration depth in bladder tissue rich with blood[8].
The charring effect at high temperatures causes sudden increased absorption of laser irradiation with subsequent disintegration, removal of tissue, and ultimate perforation.
These alternatingly slow and rapid optical and thermal events
make the Nd-YAG laser rather unsuitable as a cutting tool.
Prolonged surface heating must be avoided in transurethral
applications since this may cause a deep thermal injury
resulting in perforation and adjacent organ fistula formation.

It is surprising that more knowledge may be available
about laser light interaction with bladder tissue than the
mechanisms of electrosurgery. In the electrosurgical treatment of bladder tumors, for example, there are thermal events
in the bladder wall about which we have minimal knowledge
and limited means of controlling. Whereas, the critical advantage of the Nd-YAG laser over electrocautery maybe in the
greater depth to which the tissue is heated allowing safe and
thorough destruction of tumor cell clusters deeply imbedded
in the bladder wall. By limiting the incoming power of the
Nd-YAG laser to 40 watts in separate pulses of 1 to 3 seconds
duration to maintain tissue temperature at 60° C, the radiation
of the incoming beam is spread relatively slowly and evenly
over a broad, deep region. This permits a slow, homogeneous
heating of a large tissue volume without surface ablation[13].

DOSIMETRY

Experimental and theoretical investigations have been
performed to determine the safe and effective dosage of Nd-YAG
therapy for endoscopic treatment of bladder pathology. Since
the Nd-YAG laser produces a significant, slow, homogeneous
depth of necrosis with only slight surface blanching and
ablation, the actual extent of tissue damage may not fully
be appreciated. To assess the degree of necrosis in the
target tissue, the surgeon must have full knowledge of the
relation between irradiation dosage and observed changes
in the tissue surface.

By placing a thermocamera along the beam axis on both the
mucosal and serosal side of the bladder wall, Staehler and
associates were able to measure the temperature rise as a
function of time as the Nd-YAG laser passed through human
bladder tissue at 30 watts power with a spot diameter of 3 mm.
In water filled bladders from cystectomy specimens the maximum
temperature reached on the serosal side of the bladder wall is
50% lower than with air filled bladders. The data for water
filled bladders in contrast to air filled bladders suggest a
more gradual rise of temperature and, therefore, a safer
distribution of necrosis. For a temperature rise of 10°C,

a total energy of 120 joules (30 watts x 4 seconds) was required. For the rise of 20 to 30° C needed for coagulation
an estimate of between 200 and 300 joules via three 2 second
pulses of 40 watts each is suggested for total necrosis. To
allow for thermal equilibrium within the tissue, it is further
suggested to wait several seconds between the pulses[13].

Air-filled bladders of live rabbits were brought in contact with a loop of intestine and irradiated to obtain reliable information about the severity of penetrating radiation.
A 40 watt Nd-YAG beam 2 mm in diameter at 4 second pulses made
lesions in a bladder 1.5 mm thick to test the damage to the
adjacent intestine. A fistula was observed in the intestinal
mucosa after 2 weeks in about 20% of the cases. With an exposure time of only 2 seconds no fistulae were produced[13].

In comparison to the Nd-YAG laser the CO_2 laser at only
0.5 to 1 watt power produces a rapid rise in temperature up
to 100°C at the inner surface of the bladder wall followed
by carbonization, necrosis, and removal of a thin portion
(2-4mm) of the superficial tissue layer. The outer, serosal
layer of the bladder is relatively unaffected. During
irradiation with an Argon laser at a power of a few watts,
the thermal behavior observed is similar to that of the CO_2
except the layer of necrosis is slightly deeper. Although
the Nd-YAG laser has a deeper thermal action than that of the
CO_2 or Argon lasers, its beam intensity falls off secondary
to the scattering within the tissue and the thickness of the
bladder wall. Therefore, the applied Nd-YAG laser power on
the bladder should not be more than 45 watts to create a
mucosal surface temperature rise no greater than 90° C and a
depth of necrosis of about 3 mm. An irradiation on-time of
no more than 4 seconds should be used to achieve an irradiated
spot of about 3 mm diameter. To reach a greater depth of
necrosis, the tissue must be allowed to cool while the lesion
is irradiated at new points for short intervals of only one to
two seconds[8].

The optical properties at the bladder's mucosal surface
remain unaffected by superficial cooling with water irrigation
during Nd-YAG laser irradiation. Hence, the coagulation temperature in the deeper layers of the bladder wall is reached
without superficial tissue ablation. When white discoloration
occurs at the tissue surface, a cone of necrosis has already
reached a depth of 4-6 mm depending on the irradiation
energy[20].

CLINICAL EXPERIENCE

The Nd-YAG laser may be applied in all urologic conditions
where the applied therapy of coagulation necrosis would be useful to control bleeding and to limit tumor growth. It not only
has been adapted for endoscopic or external surgery, but also
may be coupled by an adjustable adaptor to a surgical microscope for microsurgical use.

Advantages

The advantages of the Nd-YAG laser include:
1. Precision of beam application

2. Thrombosis of small vessels
3. Reduction in bleeding
4. Rapid treatment of conditions with multiple small tumors
5. Superficial and deep coagulation of tumor tissue
6. Vaporization of tumor tissue
7. Interruption of lymphatic drainage
8. No need for general anesthesia
9. Use in out-patient surgery reduces hospitalization costs
10. Shorter operating room time
11. Post-op bladder drainage by catheter unnecessary

Disadvantages

The disadvantages of the Nd-YAG laser include:
1. Beam is too small for use in large tumors
2. Power is too low for a large volume of tissue
3. Risk of perforation and fistula from forward scattering through bladder tissue
4. Risk of eye damage to the surgeon from back scattering
5. High cost of the instrument
6. Limited exposure and education of the surgeon

INDICATIONS

Endoscopic Applications:
1. Pedunculated or sessile bladder tumors 3 cm or less in diameter
2. Stage T3 bladder tumors for palliative control of bleeding and local extension
3. Adjunctive irradiation of deep muscle bed following transurethral resection of bladder tumors greater than 3 cm in diameter to achieve homogeneous necrosis of any residual microscopic tumor cells
4. Adjunctive irradiation of the prostatic capsule following transurethral resection of carcinoma of the prostate[15]
5. Irradiation of short urethral strictures and bladder neck contractures
6. Irradiation of urethral carcinomas and condylomas

Open Surgical Applications:
1. Irradiation of condylomata of the external genitalia and urethral meatus
2. Irradiation of squamous cell carcinoma and malignant melanoma of the penis
3. Irradiation of tumor bed in solitary renal cell carcinoma or palliation for extracapsular renal tumor extension
4. Laser coagulation for hemostasis of bleeding tissue surfaces
5. Microsurgery of small anatomic or vascular lesions

CONTRAINDICATIONS

1. Nd-YAG laser is not effective for exclusive use in bladder tumors greater than 3 cm in diameter
2. Endoscopic Nd-YAG laser use to destroy bladder stones is not clinically feasible[16,17]

3. Nd-YAG laser is not useful for long urethral strictures. The Argon laser has been used successfully for
longer strictures[18]. The CO_2 laser, with its minimal
damage to adjacent tissue, may prove to be the best
modality for stricture therapy[19].

SURGICAL TECHNIQUE

In endoscopic bladder irradiation, the patient is positioned in the standard lithotomy position and given mild
intravenous sedation such as Diazepam or a short acting nar-
cotic. Intraurethral xylocaine jelly 2% may be supplemented
or a spinal block may be employed. General endotracheal anesthesia is rarely necessary. The bladder is irrigated with
saline during irradiation to wash away bleeding which would
prevent local absorption of the laser beam and weaken its
coagulating effect. The mobile fiber used with the Albarren
laser cystoscope is positioned with an irradiation gap of
only 3-5 mm at 40 watts power for 2 or 3 seconds to treat a
bladder tumor of 3 cm or less. This mobile fiber of 0.6 mm
diameter combines a high divergence of the beam at the distal
end with a very small variation of refractive index. This
achieves a higher power density of homogeneous irradiation at
the lesion while using a lower power at the proximal end[8].
Extensive laser radiation of the bladder or prostatic capsule
following transurethral electroresection of larger bladder
and prostate tumors requires observation for 2 to 3 days to
rule out secondary visceral perforation. Biopsies are taken
before and after irradiation.

External laser irradiation may be performed on obvious
lesions of the external genitalia. Local penile anesthesia
is accomplished with Xylocaine 2% injected into the neural
bundles at the base of the penis. A tourniquet is applied
around the root of the penis with a quarter inch penrose drain
and a clamp to reduce penile bleeding. A special tube with a
gas jet is incorporated in the laser handpiece to blow away
severe bleeding. Coagulation is more difficult in the presence of escaping blood due to strong absorption of laser
power, carbonization, and loss of energy. Although the tumor
may be coagulated with the Nd-YAG laser in only 3 to 5 minutes
protective goggles with side visors must be worn at all times
to prevent irreversible retinal damage from reflected laser
light. Condylomata of the urethral meatus may be exposed with
a nasal speculum or traction sutures and irradiated directly.
Condylomata of the distal urethra are best managed endoscopically. Biopsies must be taken pre-operatively[20].

ANALYSIS OF CLINICAL RESULTS

No prospective randomized trials between laser irradiation and conventional therapy are available. Until these
studies are performed, it will be very difficult to assess
the actual overall efficacy of laser technique. However,
several workers have selected their patients in such a
critical fashion that their results have proven to be encouraging.

Bladder Tumors
Hofstetter and Frank evaluated Nd-YAG laser therapy in
bladder tumors of 132 patients. Patients with different

sized bladder tumors were divided into 4 groups: (1) treated
with laser alone, (2) TUR in combination with laser, (3) TUR
plus laser coagulation and Thio Tepa, and, (4) TUR plus laser
coagulation and Mitomycin C. These four groups were compared
to a similarly composed group of patients with bladder tumors
treated with TUR alone. There was no control group treated by
intravesical chemotherapy alone. Three year survival rate with
laser treated patients approaches 70% while that for patients
treated exclusively with TUR was about 40%. Since the stages of
the tumors were comparable in both groups, it is difficult to
attribute the more favorable results in the laser group to
better patient selection[20]. Relapse rates of bladder tumors
treated with laser radiation varied between 17 and 40%. These
results compare with patients treated by TUR alone. Similarly,
the higher grade tumors in both laser and TUR treated groups had
a higher rate of recurrence.

Okada, Asaoka et al reported their experience with transurethral Nd-YAG laser treatment of 63 bladder tumors in 45
patients. Tumors were classified as small ($<$1 cm diameter) or
medium (1-3 cm diameter). They were further described as either
pedunculated or sessile. Pre-operative biopsies classified
the stage and grade of tumor. Laser technique established one
unit of irradiation as 50 watts power at 5 sec. duration or
250 joules. Each operation utilized from 5 to 50 units of
irradiation. 37 of 42 small tumors (88%) were eradicated by
laser irradiation alone; however, only 4 of 21 medium sized
tumors (19%) could be successfully treated by laser alone.
Pedunculated lesions (74%) responded more favorably to just
laser therapy than sessile tumors (31%). Grades 2 and 3 tumors
were generally treated in combination with electroresection
rather than by laser therapy alone. 3 of 23 patients who had
laser therapy alone experienced recurrence, while relapse
occurred in 8 of 22 patients undergoing combination therapy.
Since the higher grade tumors were selected for combination
therapy, this correlates with the higher rate of recurrence.
The authors found no visceral perforation, obturater nerve
reflex or significant bleeding from this treatment. Since Nd-
YAG laser therapy may be performed with local anesthesia, high
risk patients with cardiac, neurologic, or hemorrhagic diseases
may be more safely managed. The larger, high grade T2 tumors,
especially located along the anterior wall, were treated with
greater difficulty[9].

Two series from Germany summarize the experience with small
and larger bladder tumors. Hofstetter et al described the endoscopic application of the Nd-YAG laser in the treatment of 302
small tumors less than 3 cm in diameter[21]. 196 larger tumors
were treated with Nd-YAG laser irradiation after electroresection as described by Staehler[22]. They emphasized the advantages of the laser therapy as no general anesthesia, no perforation, no bleeding and shorter operative time. Their indications preferred multiple, small tumors growing diffusely
across the posterior bladder wall.

Penile Carcinoma
Hofstetter, Frank et al treated 11 patients for carcinoma
of the penis with Nd-YAG laser therapy. 7 patients had no
local relapse or metastases in 4 years. 2 patients with T1 and
T2 tumors underwent inguinal lymph node dissection in addition
to local laser therapy and have been free of tumor for 1-3 years

respectively. One patient with metastases died of his disease
and was found to have a recurrent carcinoma on the glans penis.
A patient with malignant melanoma of the glans was treated with
Nd-YAG laser but died of his disease 20 months later. No histologic evidence of residual tumor was found on the penis at
necropsy[20]. Admittedly, this small series represents only a
few anecdotal reports. Nevertheless, salvage of the penis was
achieved in seven of eleven patients without complication of
metastasis or death.

Urethral Strictures
The high recurrence rate of 20-30% occurring in the treatment of urethral stricture disease with the various reconstructive and endoscopic procedures available prompted investigations
in the use of the Nd-YAG laser[23]. Bulow et al believed that the
laser would not only cut the scar tissue but also vaporize it
and, thus, promote less adjacent tissue injury with further
scarring. Bulow used the Nd-YAG laser successfully for short
strictures of the urethra[24]; however, Rothauge demonstrated
remarkable results with the Argon laser in both short and long
urethral strictures[18]. Some of the longer strictures were managed in two stages one week apart with oral corticosteroid
therapy. Six patients out of 40 required a second laser urethrotomy after one year's follow up. As technology advances to
provide flexible fibers to transmit the CO_2 laser, the physical
properties of this laser may prove to be the most efficient for
vaporizing scar tissue and reducing recurrent formation of peri-
urethral fibrosis[19].

Prostate Cancer
Sander et al studied 5 patients who underwent TUR prostate
for carcinoma of the prostate. Nd-YAG laser irradiation was
performed as a second procedure 4 to 6 weeks later under spinal
anesthesia. The laser was operated at 50-55 watts in pulses
not exceeding 4 seconds until the entire prostatic cavity was
photocoagulated with 7000 to 13,000 joules. One of the five
patients developed urinary retention post-operatively and required catheterization. There were no perforations, bleeding
or infections. It is suggested that for patients with prostate
cancer stages $T_1 N_0 M_0$ and $T_2 N_0 M_0$ transurethral electroresection of the prostate may not be sufficient to eradicate all
microscopic disease. Radical prostatectomy with its high incidence of complications, loss of sexual function, and contra-
indication in the older age groups may be too aggressive for
many patients. Perhaps Nd-YAG laser irradiation combined with
careful transurethral electroresection offers another method of
treatment in addition to x-ray therapy[15].

CONCLUSIONS AND FUTURE CONSIDERATIONS

The use of the Nd-YAG laser for endoscopic and open surgical treatment of urologic conditions is in its embryonic
stage. Pioneers from Germany, Norway, Sweden, and Japan lead
the world in this initial experience. Hofstetter, Frank,
Staehler, and their associates are to be commended for their
superb efforts to understand the thermal events in bladder
tissue with endoscopic Nd-YAG laser irradiation. Their comparative data from tissue studies of the Nd-YAG laser, CO_2
laser and the Argon laser have provided urologists with the
fundamentals of dosimetry and safety. With this knowledge
others will be able to initiate future advances in endoscopic

research and laser engineering.

Future considerations for safer endoscopic Nd-YAG laser surgery include the use of an ultrasonic transurethral probe for constant monitoring of depth of irradiation in either the bladder or prostate[24]. Open renal surgery for hemorrhagic tumors, staghorn calculi, and partial nephrectomy deserves further investigation with the Nd-YAG laser. Although experimental disintegration of bladder stones has not yet been developed for clinical application, advanced laser technology may deliver sufficient power for transurethral or endourologic stone destruction[16]. Microsurgical application of the Nd-YAG laser on vascular, neoplastic and reconstructive conditions of the penis, testes and kidneys could stimulate an entire discipline of microurology.

The high cost of research and development in the short term must justify the savings gained with fewer hospitalizations, more ambulatory procedures, reduced blood loss, and less morbidity in the long term. In the United States federal restrictions may hamper the freedom of investigation and retard the exposure and education of laser surgeons. Hopefully, this selective process will stimulate research and clinical experience of the highest quality.

116

REFERENCES

1. R.L. Parsons, J.L. Campbell, M.W. Thomley, C.G. Butt, T.E. Gordon Jr., The Effect of the Laser on Dog Bladders: A preliminary report, J. Urol 95, 7-16 (1966)
2. H. Bulow, Present Status of Endoscopic Laser Techniques in Urology, Endoscopy 4, 240-243 (1979)
3. H. Mussiggang, Grundlagen der Urologischen Laser Chirurgie, Verh. Ber. Dtsch. Ges. Urol. 23, Tagung, S. 132, Springer, Berline, Heidelberg, New York, 1971
4. G. Nath, W. Gorisch, A. Kreitmair, P. Kiefhaber, Transmission of a powerful argon laser beam through a fiberoptic flexible gastroscope for operative gastroscopy, Endoscopy 5, 213 (1973)
5. C. Rothauge, J. Kranshaar, H.D. Noske, Einjahrige Erfahrungen mit der transurethralen Laser therapie des Harnblasentumors, Munchen Med. Wschr. 119, 593 (1977)
6. G. Staehler, W. Gorisch, A. Hofstetter, Ein Laser Zystoskop, Akt. Urol. 7, 363 (1976)
7. G. Staehler, A. Hofstetter, W. Gorisch, E. Keiditsch, M. Mussiggang, Endoscopy in Experimental Urology using an Argon Laser Bean, Endoscopy 8, 1-4 (1976)
8. A. Hofstetter, F. Frank, The Neodymium-YAG Laser in Urology, Basel: Editiones Roche, F. Hoffman - LaRoche Co. 1980
9. K. Okada, A. Hiroshi, T. Amagai, Y. Onoe, T. Kishimoto, Transurethral Nd-YAG Laser Surgery for Bladder Tumors, Urology 20, 404 (1982)
10. S. B. Lundquist, Personal Communication
11. M.S. McPhee, B. Ritchie, J. Tulip, D. Mador, R. Moore, W. H. Lakey, Segmental Irradiation of the Bladder with a Nd-YAG Laser Resectoscope, Proceedings, 4th Congress International Society of Laser Surgery, Tokyo, Chapter 10, pp. 42-45, (Nov. 24-27, 1981)
12. H. Bulow, Bulow, HGW Frohmuller, Transurethral Laser Urethrotomy in Man: Preliminary report, J. Urol. 121, 286 (1979)
13. G. Staehler, Th. Halldorsson, J. Langerholc, R. Bilgram, Endoscopic Applications of the Nd-YAG Laser in Urology: Theory, Results, Dosimetry, Urol. Res. 9, 45 (1981)
14. E. Keiditsch, J. Stern, J. Zimmerman, et al: Interruption of urinary bladder wall lymph drainage by Nd-YAG laser irradiation, in Atsumi, K., Nimsakul, M. (eds.): Laser Tokyo 1981. Tokyo, Inter. Group. Corp. 1981
15. S. Sander, H.O. Beisland, E. Fossberg, Neodymium-YAG Laser in the Treatment of Prostate Cancer, Urological Research, 10, 85-86 (1982)
16. Y. Tanahashi, K. Harada, I. Numatu, et al: The use of the laser beam in Urology, transurethral destruction of stones. J. Jpn. Soc. Laser Med. 1, 83 (1980)
17. J. Pensel, F. Frank, K. Rothenberger et al: Destruction of urinary calculi by Neodymium-YAG laser irradiation, in Atsumi, K., Nimsakul, M. (eds.) Laser Tokyo 1981. Tokyo Inter. Group Corp., 1981
18. C.F. Rothauge, Urethroscopic recanalization of urethral stenosis using argon laser, Urology 16, 158 (1980)
19. H. Bulow, Present and Future Plans for Laser Urologic Surgery, Lasers in Surgery and Medicine 1, 385 (1981)

References

20. A. Hofstetter, F. Frank, Laser Use in Urology, Chap. 8, Dixon, J.A. (ed.), Surgical Application of Lasers, Yearbook Medical Publishers, Inc. pp. 146-162, 1983
21. A. Hofstetter, F. Frank, E. Keiditsch, R. Bowering, Endoscopic Neodymium-YAG laser application for destroying bladder tumors, Eur. Urol. 7, 278 (1981)
22. G. Staehler, A. Hofstetter, Transurethral Laser irradiation of urinary bladder tumors, Eur. Urol. 5, 64 (1979)
23. E.J. Sacknoff, W.S. Kerr, Direct Vision Cold Knife Urethrotomy, J. Urol. 123, 492 (1980)
24. J. Pensel, K. Rothenberger, A. Hofstetter, Absichering der transurethralen therapie von Blasentumoren durch einen endoresikalen A. Scanner., Urologe (A) 20, 315 (1981)

CHAPTER 13

DIFFERENT LASERS IN NEUROSURGERY: A COMPARISON OF Nd:YAG AND CO_2

Peter Wolf Ascher, M.D.
Graz, Austria

DIFFERENT LASERS IN NEUROSURGERY: A COMPARISON OF ND: YAG AND CO$_2$

PETER WOLF ASCHER, M.D.
8010 Graz, Kopernikugasse 15, Graz, Austria

After of years of negative results achieved with Ruby, then CO$_2$ laser, we have simultaneously at the University of Graz and University of Munich began the clinical use of laser in neurosurgery. From each point of view the approach has been philosophically different. Using the CO$_2$ laser in Graz, we searched for indications for the use of no touch technique in neurosurgery. At wavelength 10.6 microns, the CO$_2$ laser is a relatively ineffective instrument for coagulation. On the other hand, in Munich, those working with Nd: YAG at wavelength 1.06 microns focused their efforts on coagulating highly vascularized tumors, exploiting the unique properties of the Nd: YAG. This wavelength is reflected and scattered more than absorbed. Beginning with these disparate points of view, the two institutions have gradually adopted the instruments in order to arrive at a common ground, in which each is utilized to its particular advantage. Prior to clinical evaluations, extensive laboratory experimentation has defined the affect of laser on central nervous tissue. The group in clinic Leheta and Beck, working with the Nd: YAG laser have demonstrated in many papers the tissue reaction to YAG irradiation. Similarly, the biophysical effects of CO$_2$ have been demonstrated in our laboratory and have been presented in approximately 50 scientific papers. The special applications for the CO$_2$ laser have been defined in Graz, using the instrument in combination with the operating microscope. Simultaneously, in Munich, the optical fiber uses of light YAG laser were defined and exploited. In Munich, Nd: YAG was chosen because of the presence of the MBB-AT Company which manufactured that instrument. In Graz, CO$_2$ was chosen because of the fortuitous observation of a carbon dioxide laser at the Vienese Surgical Congress. As a function of this histologic phenomenon, the two institutions explored laser from different theoretical points of view. Following initial competition the two institutions recognized the complimentary nature of their instruments and investigations, and for the past several years have colloborated on clinical and experimental studies.

In 1975, the author had been informed that his request for a combination CO$_2$- YAG laser was impossible on theoretic physical grounds. By 1981, the request was repeated, but the rejection was based on commercial projections of both manufacturers. Fortunately, a Japanese firm has been undaunted by either theoretical or commercial obstacles and will shortly go into production with a combination of carbon dioxide (30 watts) and Nd: YAG (70 watts) combination unit. This certainly represents a major advance in the development of laser surgical technique in neurological surgery. It capitalizes on the unique advantages and minimizes the particular disadvantages of each wavelength. Nevertheless, it represents only the initial steps of a new trend, basically idealized, in laser neurosurgery. Comparison of Carbon Dioxide and Nd: YAG: Both systems, one a gas and the other a solid state, develop monochromatic and, coherent and columated light. This light, upon impact with tissue, are transformed to thermal energy. Tissue reaction is a function of wavelength. Carbon dioxide, with a wavelength of 10.6 microns, is immediately absorbed by human tissue. Vaporization of intracellular water results in the explosion of the cellular structures at the surface. The Nd: YAG laser, at wavelength 1.06 microns, is less absorbed (more scattered both forward and backward. The depth of penetration proceeds slowly, by comparison, in deeper tissues are heated in more gradual fashion, allowing protein denaturation prior to cell explosion. Thus, the carbon dioxide laser is ideal for cutting and vaporization, while the Nd: YAG is best appreciated in coagulation and photo coagulation. Indications: Regardless of biophysical effect, the laser in general represents an expansion over conventional neurosurgical techniques. Conversely, when used inappropriately, neurosurgical risks are magnified. Laser

Neodymium-YAG Laser in Medicine and Surgery, Joffe, Muckerheide, and Goldman, editors

surgery is not claimed to replace conventional methods and instruments of tissue handling.

In addition, because of the relatively high expense of the instruments, economic justification requires a categorization of indications.

A. Absolute Indications
B. Relative Indications
C. No Indications

Under "absolute indications" we list those operations which are impossible or dangerous in terms of the high risk of post-operative complications by conventional means. Under "relative indications" we consider those operations which accrue to benefit the patients such as earlier mobilization, less pain, less blood loss, shorter hospitalization, lower morbidity, etc. In addition, physician benefits are considered under this category and include such considerations as shortened operative time, improved visability, improved facility. Nonindicated applications include those situations in which conventional methods are at least as good, if not superior, to laser technique.

During the period during which laser has been in routine use at the University of Graz, 10,600 operations have been performed. Of these, 680 have been considered laser indicated cases, 60 of which were "absolutely" indicated. Clinical Use: As we have indicated in our 50 papers (Ascher and Hepner), six chapters, and one book, the absolute indications include those benign, extraaxial tumors of the central nervous system, including fourth ventricle and spinal cord, which are located in neurologically sensitive areas. The more fibrous or difficult to mechanically remove, the greater the indication for laser. In many situations, surgery in these areas for these type neoplasm had heretofore been impossible. By the minimization of mechanical, thermal, and the electrical trauma to the surrounding neural and vascular structures, surgical removal has become a possibility. The thermal reaction is calculable and controllable to a limit of several microns beyond the lesion. Contact free cutting is no longer a surgeon's dream. Small tumors, up to a volume of several cubic centimeters, can be totally vaporized. A new dimension of surgery, therefore, has been inaugurated. Additionally, CO_2 laser is easily adapted to the operating microscope. The Nd: YAG laser finds its absolute indication in elderly and debilitated patients harboring highly vascularized tumors adjacent to or invading major dural sinuses. In these cases, the coagulative properties become tantamount. The surgical procedure becomes virtually bloodless and the devascularization of the tumor results in shrinkage of the neoplasm itself. Surgical removal is thus facilitated. If radical removal of the neoplasm is rendered technically impossible by invasion into the sinus, deep photocoagulation of tumor within the sinus, while sparing its protective wall, is possible. In this application, the superficial anatomical structure (sinus wall) remains in tact while the deep structure is denatured. Because of its ability to pass through an optical fiber and clear fluid media, the Nd: YAG laser becomes the instrument of choice in all intraventricular procedures.

CONCLUSION

On cumulative experience over eight years and simultaneous experience for the past two years shows that both the carbon dioxide and Nd: YAG laser systems, when used under proper indications, widen our surgical horizons. Conversely, the inappropriate use of either or both systems will offer not only surgical disadvantages but the loss of creditability of the beneficial affects of laser in neurological surgery.

122

REFERENCES:

1. Ascher, P.W., Oberbauer, R., Knoetgen, I., Holzer, P.: Vorteile und Moglichkeiten des CO_2-Lasers in der Neurochirurgie. Wien. Med. Wschr. 127(1977) 260.

2. Ascher, P.W., Oberbauer, R.W., Clarici, G., Tritthart, H.: Laserstrahl, ein modernes neurochirurgisches Instrument. IN: Neurochirurgie von Heute, Kwizda Wien (1977) 53.

3. Ascher, P.W.: Longitudinal median myelotomy with Laser. In. Neurorad. Surg., Exc. Med., Amsterdam-Oxford (1977).

4. Ascher, P.W., Oberbauer, R.W.: Gebrauch des CO_2-Lasers in der Neuro-chirurgie. In: Laser 77, ipc Science and technology press, Richmond (1977).

5. Ascher, P.W., Oberbauer, R.W., Heppner, F., Walter, G., Ingolitsch, E.: Laserbeam - a new microsrugical instrument. Proc. Int. Conf. on Lasers 1978, Spie. 1978, S. 696-699.

6. Ascher, P.W.: Der CO_2-Laser in der Neurochirurgie. Molden-Verlag Wien-Zurich (1977).

7. Ascher, P.W.: The use of the CO_2-Laser in neurosurger-. In: Laser surg., Vol. 2, Jerusalem Acad. Press, Jerusalem (1978).

8. Ascher, P.W., Ingolitsch, E., Walter, G., Oberbauer, R.: Ultrastructural findings in CNS tissue with CO_2 laser. In: Laser Surgery, Vol. 2, Jerusalem Acad. Press (1978).

9. Ascher, P.W., Heppner, F.: CO_2-Laser, a new neurosurgical instrument. Seara Med. Neurocir. 7 (1978)97-137.

10. Ascher, P.W.: Die Entiwcklung des Sharplan 791 CO_2 Lasers zum neuro-chirurgischen Instrument. Kongrebbericht, 19 Tagg. Osterr. Ges. f. Chir., EgermannWien (1979) 471-473.

11. Ascher, P.W., Ingolitsch, E., Walter, G.: Neuere histologische Unter-suchungsergebnisse nach Gebrauch des CO_2-Laser amZNS. Kongrebbericht 19.Tagg. Osterr. Ges.f.Chir., Egermann Wien (1979) 479-483.

12. Ascher, P.W.: Myelotomy with Laser. Proc. Royal Soc. Med. In Press.

13. Ascher, P.W., Heppner, F.: Clinical applications of Laser in Neuro-surgery. In: Lasers in Medicine, John Wiley and Son, Chichester, New York, Brisbane, Toronto (1981).

14. Ascher, P.W., Heppner, F.: Lasers in Medicine. Prof. Fin. "Laser di Potencia:, Proc. "Applicazioni Medichi" Florenz (1979) S. 22-28.

15. Ascher, P.W.: The Value of Recent Advances in Radiographic and Neuro-Surgical Techniques in the Removal of Spinal Canal Lesions. In: Value of Radiographic Studies in Spinal Surgery.

16. Ascher, P.W.: Newest ultrastructural findings after the use of a CO_2-Laser on CNS tissue. Acta Neurochir. Suppl. 28, Springer Verl. Wien, New York (1979) 572-581.

17. Ascher, P.W., Heppner, F.: Neurosurgical Laser Techniques. In: The

Biomedical Laser, Springer Publ., New York, Heidelberg Wien (1981).

18. Ascher, P.W.: Microsurgical Use of the CO_2-Laser in Neurosurgery. In: Microscopic and Endoscopic Surgery with the CO_2-Laser. J. Wright, Boston-Bristol-London (1982).

19. Ascher, P.W., Heppner, F.: Moglichkeiten und Grenzen des CO_2-Lasers in der Neurochirurgie. Biomed. Techn. 24 (1979) 335-336.

20. Ascher, P.W., Holzer, P.: Chirurgie der peripheren Nerven mit dem CO_2-Laser, verglichen mit herkommlichen Instrumenten. Zbl. f. Neurochir. 41 (1980) 37-40.

21. Ascher, P.W.: A Neurosurgical CO_2 Micro Laser. Digest: 7: Int. Conf. Med. & Biol. Engin., 5. Int. Conf. Med. Phys. - Binyanei Ha'voma, Jerusalem (1979) 34.

22. Ascher, P.W., Sager, W.D.: CT-Kontrollen nach Laser-Operationen. In: Derzeitige Stellung des CT in Radiologie und Klinik. Georg-Thieme-Verlag, Stuttgart (1970) 10-13.

23. Ascher, P.W.: Der CO_2-Laser in der Neurochirurgie. Forstchr. d. Med. 98 (1980) 253-254.

24. Ascher, P.W.: Laseranwendungen in der Neurochirurgie. In: Laser 79, IPC science and techn. Press. Guildford 1979.

25. Ascher, P.W., Heppner, F.: Micro Laser Surgery of the Spinal Cord. In: Laser Surg., Vol. 3, Jerusalem Acad. Press. (1980).

26. Ascher, P.W.: The CO_2-Laser, a Microsurgical Instrument. In: Laser Surg., Vol. 3, Jerusalem Acad. Press. (1980).

27. Ascher, P.W., Oberbauer, R.W., Ingolitsch, E., Walter, G.: Interaction of CO_2-Laser with the Nervour System. In: Laser Surg., Vol. 3, Jerusalem Acad. Press. (1980).

28. Ascher, P.W., Holzer, P.: Laser Surgery of Peripheral Nerves. In: Laser Surg., Vol. 3, Jerusalem Acad. Press. (1980).

29. Ascher, P.W., Clarici, G., Auer, L.: Hypophysectomy with the Laser. In: Laser Surg., Vol. 3, Jerusalem Acad. Press (1980).

30. Ascher, P.W., Lanner, G., Heppner, F.: Cortical Activity, is there some bioelectrical interference with the CO_2 Laser. In: Laser Surg. Vol. 3, Jerusalem Academic Press (1980).

31. Ascher, P.W.: Advantages and limitations of the CO_2-Laser in Neurosurgery. Proc. Int. Conf. on Lasers 1979, SPIE 122-125.

32. Ascher, P.W.: Value of Recent Advances, Using the CO_2-Laser in Neurosurgery. In Press.

33. Ascher, P.W.: Lasers in Neurosurgery (History and Development). In: Laser Tokyo 81, Inter Group Corp., Tokyo, 1981.

34. Ascher, P.W.: Early Studies in Neuro Tissue - Laser Interaction. In: Laser Neurosurgery. William & Wilkins Corp. In Press.

124

36. Ascher, P.W., Cerullo, L.: Clinical Results of Laser Use in Neurosurgery. In: Surgical Application. In Press.

37. Ascher, P.W.: Comparison of different Laser Systems in Neurosurgery.
In: Congress Proceedings. In Press.

38. Ascher, P.W.: Absolute Indikationen fur den Einstaz des CO_2-und
Neodym-YAG-Lasers. Fortschritte der Medizin. In Press.

39. Ascher, P.W., Walter, G.F., Ingolitsch, E.: The effect of Carbon-
dioxide-and Neodymium-YAG lasers on the central and peripheral nervous
system, cerebral blood vessels and the Pituitary gland. In Press.

40. Fox, J.L., Hayes, J.R., Stein, M.N.: The effects of laser radiation on
intracranial structures. In: Abstr. 1st Ann. Biomed. Laser Conf.,
Boston (1965).

41. Heppner, F., Ascher, P.W.: Uber den Einsatz des Laserskalpells in der
Neurochirurgie. Act. Med. Techn. 24 (1976) 424.

42. Heppner, F., Ascher, P.W.: Hirnoperationen mit dem CO_2-Laser. Melsunger
Nachr. Bd. 51/II, Suppl. (1977)121-122.

43. Heppner, F., Ascher, P.W. Erste Versuche mit dem Laserstrahl in der
Behandlung neurochirurgischer Erkrankungen. Zbl. f. Neurochir. 38
(1977) 77.

44. Heppner, F., Ascher, P.W.: Operationen am Hirn und Ruckenmark mit dem
Sharplan 791 CO_2-Laser. Acta chir Austriaca 2 (1977) 32.

45. Heppner, F., Ascher, P.W.: Experiences with the CO_2-Laser during
treatment of lesions of central and peripheral nervous system. J.
Neurosurg. Submitted for publication.

46. Heppner, F.: Neurochirurgische Operationen mit dem CO_2-Laser. Neuro-
logia et Psychiatria 1,1 (1978) 9-13.

47. Heppner, F.: Behandlung von Mittellinien-Lasionen des gehirns mit
dem CO_2-Laser. Kongress-Bericht Osterr. Chir. Kongress 1978, 19.
Tagg. Vlg. Egermann, Wien (1979) 21-30.

48. Heppner, F., Clarici, G.: The operative approach to lipomas of the
Corpus Callosum. Neurochirurgia 22 (1979)3, 77-81.

49. Heppner, F.: The Laser Scalpel on the Nervous System. In: J. Kaplan:
Laser Surgery II. Jerusalem. Academic Press (1978) 79ff.

50. Heppner, F.: Erfahrungen mit dem CO_2-Laser in der Chirurgie des Nerven-
systems. Abl. Neurochir. 40 (1979) 297-304.

51. Heppner, F.: Nerere Technologien im Einsatz gegen hirneigene bosartige
Geswulste. Vortrag, gehalten 10.0kt. 1980, Osterr, Akademie der Wiss.
In Press.

52. Heppner, F.: CO_2-Laser Surgery of the Spinal Cord. In: Laser Surg.
Vol. 3, Jerusalem Acad. Press, 1980.

53. Heppner, F.: Der Laser in der Neurochirurgie. Buchbeitrag "Der Laser",
hrsg. K. Dinstl, P.L. Fischer, Springer-Verlag Berlin-Heidelberg- New
York (1981) 143.

54. Heppner, F.: New Technologies to Combat Malignant Tumours of the Brain. Anticancer Research 2 (1982) 101-110.

55. Heppner, F.: The CO_2-Laser in Neurosurgery. In: Internat. Advances in Surgical Oncology V. Alan Liss, Inc., New York (1982).

56. Heppner, F.: Lasers in Neurosurgery and their Forerunners. In: New Frontiers in Laser Surgery and Medicine, Buchbeitrag. In Press.

57. Heppner, F.: Der medizinische Laser und sein Vorlaufer. In Press.

58. Heppner, F.: Die Heilende Hitze. Fortschr. der Medizin (1983), Vortrag gehalten 4. Nov. 1982. 1. Tagg. der Deutschen Gesellschaft fur Lasermedizin, Munchen.

CHAPTER 14

PRESENT APPLICATIONS OF THE Nd:YAG LASER IN NEUROSURGERY

Victor Aldo Fasano
Institute of Neurosurgery
University of Turin
Torino, Italy

PRESENT APPLICATIONS OF THE Nd:YAG LASER IN NEUROSURGERY

VICTOR ALDO FASANO
Institute of Neurosurgery, University of Turin, via Cherasco 15,
10126 Torino, Italy.

There are some experimental data on the biological effects of the Nd:YAG laser. The main characteristics are the low absorption and high scattering, in the brain with a beam diameter of 2.4-3.6 mm the depth of the lesion is 3.78 mm and the lateral extension is 6.8 mm (Beck, 1979)[1]. In small vessels a complete occlusion by endovascular thrombosis can be achieved using laser (Boergen, 1981)[2]. In large vessels a diffuse shrinkage of the walls can be obtained with Nd:YAG irradiation (Gorisch, 1977)[8]. The shrinkage, even without obliteration of the lumen, increases other vessel-sealing effects through adherence of coagulated erythrocyte aggregations to the vessel walls and subsequent thrombus formation[2].

Our experience on the Nd:YAG laser is referred to the tumoral surgery (cerebral tumors, spinal tumors, intraventricular tumors)[4,6,7] and the vascular surgery (arteriovenous malformations)[3,5].

We have used since 1980 the Nd:YAG laser in neurosurgery. Our case studies include 80 surgical cases: 60 cerebral tumors, 12 vascular malformations, and 8 spinal cord tumors. We discuss here the surgical indications in various pathologies.

The main problems are: the hemostatic effect, the modifications of the compactness of the tissue, the consequences on the nervous tissue of the thermic spreading; the characteristics of the functional damage on nervous tissue; and the delayed effects.

We use the Nd:YAG laser in vascularized tumors mostly to achieve hemostasis which is limited to vessels of 1.5-2 mm. It is mostly a diffuse arteriolar bleeding that is controlled by Nd:YAG laser, but it is important to point out that the Nd:YAG cannot produce a complete hemostasis of the mass.

The reduction in compactness of the tissue by Nd:YAG irradiation has been observed to facilitate the demolition of the bulk of the tumor.

The main problem in the use of the Nd:YAG laser is the thermic spreading on the surrounding tissues. Staelher (1980) studied the thermic damage on an adjacent organ (intestine loop in immediate contact with the bladder at the site where the irradiation takes place)[9]. With a power of 40 watts, a spot diameter of 2 mm and an exposure time of 4 seconds a lesion was observed in intestinal mucosa in about 20% of the cases. No thermic effects on adjacent organs are observed if the applied power level is not higher than 40 watts and the exposure time not longer than 2 seconds. Sundt (1983)[10] by recording the temperature at various depths from the cortical surface, determined that a maximum of 15-20 watts for 8 seconds could be safely applied to cat cortex in vivo. These data are not absolute, particularly when the Nd:YAG is used free-hand. Our recent research on a comparative study of lesions produced by Nd:YAG with conventional histology, ultrastructural study and autoradiography shows that the cellular damage is greater than the damage visible under light microscope. Besides the different effects produced on the vessel walls make possible the extension of the intravascular thrombosis as a consequence of the irradiation producing a further extension of the lesion.

We underline the usefulness of the laser in neurosurgery is essentially linked to the limitation of its damage effects; it must also be used in very

© 1983 by Elsevier Science Publishing Co., Inc.
Neodymium-YAG Laser in Medicine and Surgery, Joffe, Muckerheide, and Goldman, editors

restricted areas. For these reasons the practical use of the Nd:YAG shows some limitation in comparison with CO_2 laser.

In the tumoral implants on the dura mater (falx meningiomas, basal meningiomas, parasagittal meningiomas, spinal cord meningiomas) the Nd:YAG laser produces a complete hemostasis of the infiltrated dura and permits reduction of recurrences because of the deeper penetration.

In parasagittal meningiomas the Nd:YAG laser can be used when the tumor implant occludes the venous sinus; if the sinus is patent the risk of a progressive thrombosis reduces the usefulness of this method.

Because of the low absorption in acqueous media Nd:YAG has been used for the hemostasis of the intraventricular tumors (choroid plexus papillomas, intraventricular meningiomas).

In the treatment of arteriovenous malformations the Nd:YAG laser allows a complete extirpation with reduced blood losses and minimal manipulation of the surrounding tissues. Veins are occluded easily. In the thin feeding arteries the shrinkage produced by the laser is followed rapidly by complete obliteration of the lumen. In larger and thicker vessels the occlusion is delayed by thrombosis. The present indications are small arteriovenous malformation in critical areas of the brain.

In medium sized saccular aneurysms the Nd:YAG laser cannot be used because of the risk of the extension of the thrombosis to the parent artery. The Nd:YAG laser could be useful to treat giant aneurysms.

REFERENCES

1. Beck,O.J., Wilske,J., Schonberger,J.L., Gorisch,W.,(1979). Tissue Changes Following Application of Lasers to the Rabbit Brain. Results with CO_2 and Neodymium-YAG lasers. Neurosurg.Rev.,1,31-36.

2. Boergen,K.P., Birngruber,R., Hillenkamp,F.(1981). Laser induced endovascular thrombosis as a possibility of selective vessel closure. Ophthalmic Res.,13,139-150.

3. Fasano,V.A.(1981). The Treatment of vascular malformations of the brain with laser sources. Lasers in Surgery and Medicine,1,347-356.

4. Fasano,V.A.,Benech,F.,Ponzio,R.M.(1982). Observation on the Simultaneous Use of CO_2 and Nd:YAG Lasers in Neurosurgery. Lasers in Surgery and Medicine,2,155-162.

5. Fasano,V.A., Urciuoli,R., Ponzio,R.M.(1982). Photocoagulation of Cerebral Arterio-venous malformations and Arterial Aneurysms with the Neodymium: Yttrium-Aluminum-Garnet or Argon laser. Preliminary results in Twelve Patients. Neurosurg.,11,754-760.

6. Fasano,V.A., Lombard,G.F., Ponzio,R.M.(1983). Preliminary Experiences with the Use of Three Lasers (CO_2,Nd:YAG,Argon) in Some Posterior Fossa Tumors in Childhood. Child's Brain,10,26-38.

7. Fasano,V.A.(1983). Preliminary Research on the use of different laser sources on the wall of the vessels in Rabbits. In press.

8. Gorisch,W.(1978). Temperature Measurements of isolated mesenteric blood Vessels of Rabbit during laser irradiation. Kaplan,I.(ed.) Jerusalem, Laser Surgery II pp 202-207.

9. Staehler,G., Halldorsson,T., Langerholc,J., Bilgram,R.(1980). Dosimetry for Neodymium:YAG Laser Applications in Urology. Lasers in Surgery and Medicine,1,191-197.

10. Wharen,R.E., Anderson,R.E., Sundt,T.M.(1983). The Nd:YAG Laser: An Evaluation of its Effects on Normal Brain and Ita Applicability in the Resection of Cerebral Arterio-venous Malformations. Proceedings: The American Association of Neurological Surgeon,Washington,pp 63-64.

CHAPTER 15

Nd:YAG LASER IN NEUROSURGERY

K. K. Jain, M.D.
Los Angeles, California

132

ND-YAG LASER IN MICRONEUROSURGERY

K. K. JAIN, M.D.
Los Angeles, California

INTRODUCTION

Since the introduction of lasers in neurosurgery attention has been
focussed mainly on the CO_2 laser. Mussigang (16) in 1974, was the first
to use Nd:YAG laser in experimental surgery. The first application in
neurosurgery was made by Beck (1) in Munich, Germany in 1976. Jain, also
working in Munich, started to use this laser for microvascular reconstructive surgery in 1978 (9). Now neurosurgeons in Japan are using it
clinically (19) and there is increasing interest in this laser in U.S.A.

EQUIPMENT

The author has used MEDILAS Type 2 laser (Messerschmitt-Bolkow-Blohm,
Munich, Germany) with a 600 micron core fiberoptic delivery system and
a handpiece with focussing lenses. The microadopter is not yet available
commercially. For freehand surgery under the operating microscope the
quartz fiber can be introduced into a handheld suction tube. A 4-channel
endoscope (ventriculoscope) which carries the laser fiber, fiberoptic
illumination, suction and biopsy instruments is also available. For microvascular procedures the laser handpiece is held by a micromanipulator.
For eye protection either special glasses or a special filter is used over
the objective lens of the microscope.

TISSUE EFFECTS OF ND:YAG LASER

Beck (3) has compared the effects of Nd:YAG and CO_2 lasers on the
rabbit brain. In contrast to CO_2 laser which produces discrete lesions,
Nd:YAG beam penetrates deeper into the brain tissue. There is diffuse
necrosis and edema zone extends wider. There is heat damage in tissue
areas with no visible damage in the acute stage. The effect is more
pronounced in vascular areas of the brain. Leheta and Gorisch (14) have
studied comparative effect on blood vessels of Argon and Nd:YAG lasers.
They defined the optical parameters for Nd:YAG coagulation as:

Power. . . . . 40 watts
Beam diameter. . . . . . 7-3.5 mm.
Power density(W/cm^2) . . 100-400
Time . . . . 10 sec.

Vessels up to 5 mm. in diameter could be coagulated with these parameters.
There was, however, considerable thermal damage to the surrounding tissues.
This laser is not suitable for use over critical areas of the brain. The
penetration is deeper than that by CO_2 and Argon lasers and there is more
tissue scatter (18). These characteristics have some advantages in the
surgery of vascular meningiomas. The tumor, after exposure to Nd:YAG laser,
shrinks and is reduced in vascularity. Due to scatter the size of the
lesion is larger and heat diffusion is more rapid. For ablation of
meningiomas power settings of 60-80 watts are required.

Nd:YAG laser induces vessel closure by shrinking the collagen from
the heat generated (7). For microvascular repair the parameters used are:

Power $17^{\pm} 2$ watts for arteries
                         $6^{\pm} 1$ watts for veins
Beam diameter   0.2-0.5 mm.
Time   0.05-0.1 sec.

Power density alone used as a guide is not reliable as time is the critical
factor. It is safer to use higher power for a shorter time than a low
power for a longer time. There is more tissue damage in the latter

combination.

The mechanism of closure of holes in the arteries is by contraction of collagen fibers. Vessel anastomosis is achieved by welding of collagen in the media due to physico-chemical changes as a heat effect. This is strong enough to withstand the force of pulsatile blood flow (10). The author has not observed any effects on the surrounding tissues during laser microvascular surgery as the laser spot size is less than the vessel diameter and the laser beam does not come in contact with other tissues. The heat produced by laser application is absorbed and dissipated in the blood vessel.

ND:YAG LASER AS A COAGULATING TOOL

Coagulation is an important manoeuvre during neurosurgery and bipolar coagulation has held an unchallenged place for this for several years. Various authors have compared electrocoagulation with laser coagulation (13,20,21). The advantages of Nd:YAG laser coagulation over bipolar coagulation can be summarized as follows (12).
1. There is no tissue contact with forceps and no possibility of the forceps sticking to the vessel.
2. There is no mechanical trauma to the vessel wall from pinching effect of the forceps.
3. No lesions in surrounding tissues as occur with leakage of electric current.
4. Time and intensity of heat application to the tissues can be controlled more precisely.
5. It is possible to occlude a vessel without producing thrombus.
6. It is effective for hemostasis in a patient with hemophilia.

The major disadvantage is that Nd:YAG laser is ineffective in a pool of blood. A bleeding vessel has to be held with instruments and the blood has to be suctioned out before laser can be applied to the vessel.

INDICATIONS FOR USE OF ND:YAG LASER IN NEUROSURGERY

These can be summarized as follows:
1. Microvascular surgery: Repair of blood vessels
                            Sutureless anastomosis
2. Vascular anomalies of CNS: Intracranial aneurysms
                              AVM's of CNS
3. Meningiomas
4. Hydrocephalus: Ventriculoscopy and coagulation of choroid plexus
                  Third ventriculostomy

TECHNIQUE AND DISCUSSION OF USES OF ND:YAG LASER

Prior to clinical use the surgeon should receive instruction and practice the use of Nd:YAG laser in laboratory animals. Instructions are provided in the Handbook of Laser Neurosurgery (12).

Repair of Blood Vessels

Blood vessels may be injured during surgery of brain tumors. In case of small vessels (diameter less than 1 mm.) repair is either tedious or impractical by suture technique. Sometimes the vessel is sacrificed by coagulation or ligation to stop the hemorrhage. With laser technique it is possible to repair holes and lacerations in arteries as small as 0.5 mm. in diameter with minimal stenosis and preservation of vessel patency.(8) Technique for repair of a hole in an artery in a tumor bed is shown in Fig. 1.

134

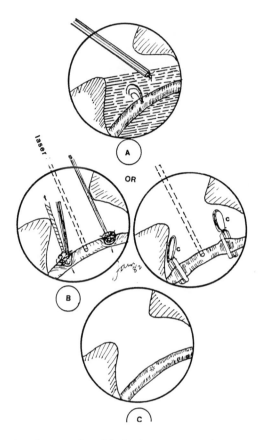

Fig. 1. Repair of hole in an artery in tumor
bed. A. Suction blood to identify the hole.
B. Try temporary arrest of hemorrhage by press-
ing artery with cottonoid strips under a forceps (f) in one hand and a microsuction (s) in
the other. Then apply Nd:YAG laser to the hole
to be repaired. Or if the pressure on the vessel
is not enough, apply two clips(c) and then lase
the hole. C. The hole is sealed and the blood
flow has resumed in the artery.

Sutureless Anastomosis

In microvascular surgery the standard method for performing arterial
anastomosis is by suture technique. The anastomosis may be end-to-end or
end-to-side. Various sutureless techniques have been evaluated including
tissue adhesives, PVP tubes and thermovascular anastomosis (12) but found
to be unsatisfactory. CO_2 laser, despite the claims by some, cannot be
used in vessel welding as it does not penetrate tissues. Anastomosis
performed with Argon laser has poor tensile strength. Argon penetration
in tissues is less than that of Nd:YAG laser and heat induced changes in
the vessel media are less than in the case of Nd:YAG laser.

End-to-end anastomosis is required for repairing accidental severing of arteries and occasionally for cerebral revascularization. The steps of the procedure are shown in Fig. 2. Vessels ranging in diameter from 0.5 to 1 mm can be anastomosed with this technique. It is not necessary to use a micro-balloon catheter but it facilitates the approximation of the vessels and prevents stenosis at the site of anastomosis. The advantages of this technique over the conventional suture anastomosis are:
1. It is faster. It takes less than 3 minutes compared to an average of 10 minutes for suture anastomosis using 8 sutures.
2. There is no trauma to the vessel wall from repeated punctures with the needle.
3. No foreign body (suture) is left in the vessel wall.
4. The patency rates are as high as 98%.
5. The results of the procedure are more consistent even though performed by different surgeons of varying degrees of manual dexterity.

There should be no complications with this procedure if proper precautions are taken. Laser beam does not penetrate to the intima. The intima reconstitutes over the site of anastomosis within a week following the procedure.

End-to-side anastomosis is usually done for extra-intracranial bypass surgery in cerebrovascular occlusive disease. The steps of this procedure are shown in Fig. 3 (11). No balloon catheter is required. The most commonly performed procedure is superficial temporal artery to middle cerebral artery anastomosis. Superficial temporal to superior cerebellar artery anastomosis for vertebral-basilar insufficiency is technically more difficult due to the site of anastomosis being at depth. This is where laser technique has an advantage as it can be performed with equal ease at depth as at the surface of the brain.

At present this is the only way to use Nd:YAG laser to achieve end-to-side anastomosis. Yahr and Strully (22) published a paper with the title "Blood Vessel Anastomosis by Laser". They used tissue adhesives to glue two arteries and used Nd:YAG laser merely to punch a hole through. Sutures were used to close the end of one of the arteries. Experiments were done on carotid arteries of the dog without microsurgical techniques. These methods were never established although frequently quoted in literature as example of first sutureless laser anastomosis of blood vessels!

VASCULAR ANOMALIES OF CNS

Arteriovenous Malformations (AVM). Beck (1) was first to extirpate an AVM with Nd:YAG laser. More recently Fassano (4,5) has published his experience on this subject. The AVM has to be exposed and the feeders identified to apply laser. The results are comparable to non-laser microsurgical procedures for this lesion. The advantage of Nd:YAG laser is in treatment of small deep seated AVM's using microstereotactic approach. This could be a safer alternative to less available forms of radiation such as Gamma knife or Proton beam.

Intracranial Aneurysms. Maira et al (15) reported their experiences with experimental aneurysms using Argon laser and Fassano (4) has used Nd:YAG laser for treating intracranial aneurysms in 5 patients. In only one case was the aneurysm completely obliterated. In view of excellent results obtained by current microsurgical techniques used in aneurysm surgery the propriety of use of laser is questioned. Nd:YAG laser applied to the fundus of an aneurysm may cause rupture of the sac. There is not enough collagen in the wall of the fundus to achieve laser induced contracture and obliteration of the sac. Based on my experience with use of Nd:YAG laser on experimental aneurysms and clinical aneurysm surgery I

136

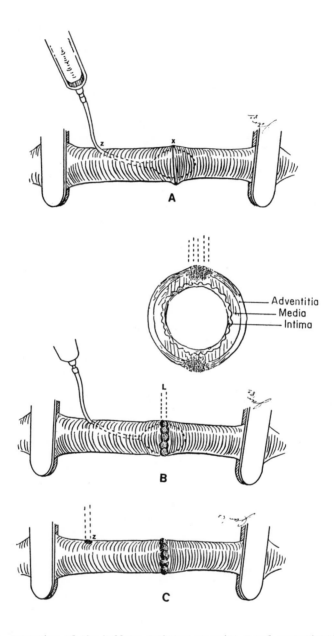

Fig.2-A. Insertion of the balloon catheter at point Z and approximation of
the two arteries at point X. The balloon is inflated. B. Anastomosis being
performed by laser beam (L). Cross section of the artery shows fusion of
the collagen of the media. C. The anastomosis is complete. The catheter
is withdrawn and the site of catheter insertion (Z) is being repaired with
laser.

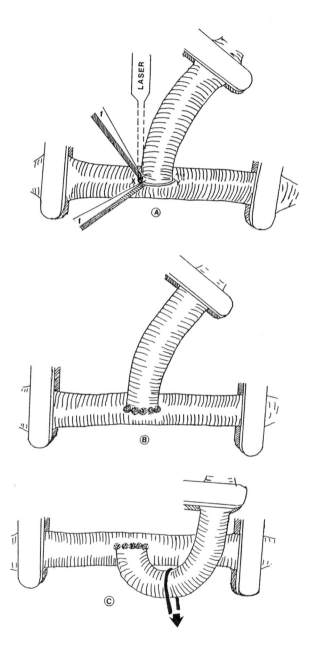

Fig.3. End-to-side anastomosis. The first spot to be fused (X) is between
the two forceps (f). B. Completed anastomosis on one side. C. The artery
loop is retracted (arrow) to expose the other side which is lased to
complete the anastomosis.

suggest that the use of Nd:YAG laser be confined to the following indications (12).
1. To obliterate small intact blebs (aneurysms?) 1-2 mm. in diameter found
    incidentally during intracranial surgery.
2. To narrow the wide neck of an aneurysm prior to placing a clip.
3. To reduce the vessel diameter in aneurysmal dilatation of an artery by
    circumferential application of laser.

The use of Nd:YAG laser is safer than the use of bipolar coagulation
in these situations as it does not carry the risk of the forceps sticking
to the aneurysm. Further refinements will have to be made in laser techniques before the current methods of aneurysm surgery can be challenged.
If an aneurysm has to be exposed surgically and is suitable for clipping
it should be clipped.

MENINGIOMAS

Nd:YAG laser is particularly useful in surgery of vascular and infiltrating meningiomas of the cranial cavity. Particular indications for the
use of this laser in this type of lesion are as follows:
1. Radiation of a large vascular meningioma prior to excision with CO_2
    laser or the simultaneous use of these two lasers (6). The tumor
    vascularity and blood loss are reduced. Retraction of tumor from the
    surrounding brain due to shrinking facilitates dissection of the tumor.
2. Meningiomas penetrating dural sinuses. Beck (1) has used Nd:YAG laser
    to radiate the residual meningioma penetrating dural venous sinuses.
    The tumor bulging into the venous sinus is destroyed by the penetrating
    heat and is eventually reduced in bulk. This obviates the need for
    sinuplasty.
3. Meningiomas infiltrating the base of skull and meningioma-en-plaque can
    be destroyed by radiation with Nd:YAG laser.
4. Intraventricular meningiomas can be ablated using Nd:YAG laser endo-
    scopic technique (2).

Advantages of Laser Technique in Surgery of Meningiomas are:

  i.   reduced blood loss
 ii.   no need for retraction of brain
iii.   reduced postoperative cerebral edema
 iv.   reduced incidence of postoperative hematoma at site of tumor
       excision
  v.   reduced recurrence

HYDROCEPHALUS

Coagulation of the choroid plexus via a Nd:YAG laser endoscope (ventriculoscope) is a potentially useful procedure to cut down CSF production and
can also be used to ablate choroid plexus papillomas.
Third ventriculostomy can be performed using Nd:YAG laser fiber in a suction
tube inserted via a small skull trephine hole. A perforation is made with
the laser in the lamina terminalis and into the cisterna interpeduncularis
(12). Nd:YAG laser can be effective in presence of CSF and in the above
two situations this is an advantage over the CO_2 laser.

LASER SAFETY

Nd:YAG laser surgery requires general safety measures for laser
surgery and the surgeon must study and follow the precautions recommended (12).

During intracranial surgery care should be taken not to expose vital

areas of the brain to this laser because of its tissue penetrating properties. This laser is not suitable for work at tumor-brain interphase where
CO_2 laser with its low tissue penetration is safer.

In microvascular work extreme care should be taken in calibrating the
laser power as higher powers than what is necessary may do irreparable
damage to the vessel. The absorption of laser energy is intensified if
arterial blood becomes darker or if there is discoloration of the vessel
wall from a previous laser application. It is important that blood vessel
anastomosis be achieved at first attempt. An improperly done anastomosis
cannot be redone with this laser.

Black sutures should not be exposed to this laser as they will
disrupt. White or light green colored sutures are safer from effects of
this laser in low intensities.

FUTURE OF ND:YAG LASER IN NEUROSURGERY

I predict useful advances in the following areas in the next decade.

1. Automation and refinement in sutureless laser microvascular anastomosis
   techniques. It will be possible to anastomose arteries less than 0.5 mm
   in diameter in less than a minute. The laser power in such a system
   would be automatically adjusted by a color sensor according to the
   hemoglobin content of the blood, state of oxygenation of the blood
   and vascularity of the arterial wall. This technique will open up the
   possibility of revascularization of critical areas of the brain and the
   spinal cord. Even the blood supply to the cranial nerves can be
   improved. According to Prof. U. Fisch of Zurich (personal communication), who has performed revascularization procedures of the ischemic
   auditory nerve for deafness, laser anastomosis of small arteries would
   be very helpful.
2. Nd:YAG laser catheter techniques. Argon laser catheters have been
   used for producing arterial occlusion in experimental animals (17).
   Similar catheters with Nd:YAG laser can be used to approach intracranial vascular lesions such as aneurysms to obliterate them without
   the need for craniotomy.
3. Experimental nerve suture. Peripheral nerve suture has been performed
   by approximating two nerves with a drop of blood in between and
   exposing to Nd:YAG laser. This technique merits further evaluation.
4. Computerized Automated Micromanipulative Surgery. Nd:YAG laser would
   be a component of such a system of surgery. The laser beam is easier
   to micromanipulate than solid instruments. Different lasers such as
   CO_2, Argon, and Nd:YAG would have the possibility to be applied
   through a common delivery system.

REFERENCES

1. O.J. Beck, The Use of Nd:YAG and CO_2 laser in neurosurgery, Neurosurg
   Rev 3:261,(1980).
2. O.J. Beck, Selective laser endoscopic coagulation of the choroid
   plexus - A method to be considered in treating hydrocephalus? In
   Kaplan I (ed) Laser Surgery, Vol III-Part II. (Jerusalem, Academic
   Press, (1979) p. 75.
3. O.J. Beck, J. Wilski, J. L. Schonberger, Tissue changes following
   application of lasers to the rabbit brain, Neurosurg Rev 1:31, (1979).
4. V.A. Fassano, R. Urciuoli, R.M. Ponzio, Photocoagulation of cerebral
   arteriovenous malformations and arterial aneurysms with Neodymium:YAG
   or Argon laser, Neurosurg 11:754, (1982).
5. V.A. Fassano, The Treatment of vascular malformations of the brain with

laser source. Lasers in Surg & Med 1:347, (1981)

6. V.A. Fassano, F. Benech, R.M. Ponzio, Observations on the Simultaneous Use of CO$_2$ and Nd:YAG lasers in neurosurgery. Lasers in Surg & Med, 2:155, (1982).

7. W. Gorisch, K.P. Boergen, Heat Induced Contraction of Blood Vessels, Lasers in Surg & Med 2:1, (1982).

8. K.K. Jain, W. Gorisch, Repair of Small Blood Vessels with Nd:YAG laser. Surgery 85:684, (1979).

9. K.K. Jain, W. Gorisch, Microvascular repair with Neodymium-YAG laser. Acta Neurochir (suppl) 28: 260, (1979).

10. K.K. Jain, Sutureless microvascular anastomosis with Neodymium-YAG laser, J. Microsurg. 1:436, (1980).

11. K.K. Jain, Sutureless end-to-side microvascular anastomosis using Neo-dymium-YAG laser. Vascular Surg. 17:1983 (July-August).

12. K.K. Jain, Handbook of Laser Neurosurgery, (Charles C. Thomas, Spring-field, Illinois, 1983).

13. E. Kleidtisch, A. Hoffstetter, K. Rothenberger et al, Comparative Morphological Investigations of the Effects of the Neodymium-YAG laser and electrocoagulation in experimental animal research, in J.H. Bellina (ed) Gynecologic Laser Surgery (Plenum Publishing Corporation, New York, 1981).

14. F. Leheta, W. Gorisch, Coagulation of Blood Vessels by Argon ion and Nd:YAG laser radiation in I Kaplan (ed) Laser Surgery (Vol 1) (Academic Press, Jerusalem, 1976) p. 178.

15. G. Maira, G. Mohn, A. Panisset, Laser photocoagulation for treatment of experimental aneurysms, J. Microsurg. 1:137, (1979).

16. H. Mussigang, W. Rother, Neodymium-YAG laser as an operative instrument in experimental surgery, Munch Med Wochenschr, 116:937, (1974).

17. G.V. O'Reilly, V.M. Colucci, D.G. Astorian, Transcatheter fiberoptic laser coagulation of blood vessels. Radiology 142:777, (1982).

18. W.W. Rother, Th. Halldorsson, J. Langerhoic, Present Status of Nd:YAG laser in endoscopy and surgery in I Kaplan (ed) Laser Surgery (Vol II), (Academic Press, Jerusalem, 1978) p. 211.

19. J. Takeuchi, H. Handa, W. Taki, The Nd:YAG laser in neurological surgery. Surg Neurol 18:140, (1982).

20. T. Takizawa, Comparison between laser surgical unit and the electro-surgical unit. Neurol Med Chir (Tokyo) 17:95, (1977).

21. B. Vallfors, Coagulation in Neurosurgery, Acta Neurochir 55:29, (1980).

22. W.Z. Yahr, K.J. Strully, Blood vessel Anastomosis by Laser and other Biomedical Applications, JAAMI 1:28, (1966).

CHAPTER 16

Nd:YAG LASER IN NEUROSURGERY

Principal Author:

Leonard P. Burke, M.D.
University Neurosurgeons, Inc.
Chicago, Illinois

Nd: YAG LASER IN NEUROSURGERY

LEONARD P. BURKE, M.D., RICHARD A. ROVIN, M.D., L.J. CERULLO, M.D.
J.T. BROWN, M.D. AND JOSEPH PETRONIO, M.D.

Histologic changes following laser irradiation were evaluated in the rat cerebral cortex. Each hemisphere was lesioned using either CO_2 or Nd: YAG laser in a focused mode, with single pulse application of either 0.1 or 0.5 seconds. Because the CO_2 laser has a smaller spot size (0.4 mm) compared to the Nd: YAG laser (1.5 mm), the power output was adjusted to result in similar power densities[1] of the two laser sources. Three power densities were evaluated, and the animals were sacrificed at two weeks, one week, or immediately. Specimens were examined by light microscopy using rutin stains.

The CO_2 laser produced a sharply demarcated lesion on the cortex measuring 0.75 to 1.00 mm in diameter, with mildly elevated borders and minimal carbonization of the crater. The lesion was frequently accompanied by bleeding at the surface. The lesion produced by the Nd: YAG laser was approximately twice as large as that noted with the CO_2 laser, though this was variable. There was no central cavity noted, except at higher power densities. On the other hand, there was more carbonization and more mounding with the Nd: YAG lesions.

On coronal section, each laser produced characteristic histologic lesions, the size and shape of which were dependent upon the power and exposure time. Regardless of the laser source, three distinct zones were always noted and have previously been described.[2]

Under low power, the CO_2 (Fig. 1) lesion was a shallow depression, measuring approximately 0.8 mm in depth. At higher output power and longer exposure, the CO_2 lesions became cone shaped with the depth being dependent on both variables but more on time.

The lesions produced by Nd: YAG laser (Fig. 2) were hemispheroidal in shape, with the width and depth dependent on the power and exposure time. Unlike the CO_2 lesions, however, the depth of the Nd: YAG lesion appeared more dependent on power output than length of exposure. The Nd: YAG lesions were consistently wider and deeper than those produced by the CO_2 laser at the lower output powers. At the highest power densities, however, the Nd: YAG lesions extended less deep but wider than the CO_2 laser. At equal power density, the histologically defined zones were larger with the YAG than with the CO_2.

When the specimens were examined immediately after lesioning intact neurons were noted in all three zones with minimal eosinophilia noted. Toward the periphery of the lesions, more eosinophilc neurons were noted with the YAG lesion than the CO_2. Extravasated red blood cells were noted in both lesions but appeared more numerous with the Nd: YAG lesions.

In the specimens which survived one week following lesioning, all lesions demonstrated numerous inflammatory cells with influx of macrophages at the periphery and center of all the lesions. Neurons at the border of the lesions had become more eosinophilic and this was more notable with the YAG lesion.

By the end of two weeks, the inflammatory response had diminished, with a greater number of macrophages being present in all lesions, some of which contained hemosiderin. Central cavitation was noted, the appearance of which resembled that of infarction. There was no essential difference except in shape between the two types of lesions.

© 1983 by Elsevier Science Publishing Co., Inc.
Neodymium-YAG Laser in Medicine and Surgery, Joffe, Muckerheide, and Goldman, editors

In summary, it appears that the effect of Nd: YAG and CO_2 on rat cerebral tissue was essentially the same, except for the difference in shape and size of the lesions caused by the two laser sources. At lower powers, Nd: YAG lesions are consistently deeper and wider, while at higher powers the CO_2 lesion was consistently narrower and much deeper. The basic cellular reactions appeared similar.

Stimulated but what appeared to be viable neurons both within and at the margins of the lesions created by both laser sources, we initiated a study to evaluate the physiochemical interaction of laser and neural tissue. A technique for catecholamine histofluorescence, described by De La Torre,[3] was employed. The series of animals were used to compare Nd: YAG and CO_2 lesions of identical power densities and radiant exposures in acute and chronic (one month) preparations.

While both lasers generate lesions that are characterized by a "central zone" of coagulation necrosis and well demarcated borders, there are subtle differences between the lasers with respect to the acute (less than one hour) response of the catecholamine terminal.

In the Nd: YAG lesions, the central coagulation was surrounded by a homogenous granular zone, devoid of catecholamine terminals, though still appearing viable by H and E stains. Catecholamine fibers abruptly end at the lateral margins of this granular zone, extending the physiologic size of the lesion by a factor of .3. By contrast in the CO_2 lesions catecholamine terminals directly abut the central coagulum, and some terminals actually extend within the lesion itself. After 3 days, dramatic changes in the catecholamine fiber patterns occur in Nd: YAG lesion. The catecholamine terminals now extend directly to the margins of the lesion, where there is no evidence of a granular zone. The chronic (one month) preparation continued to show catecholamine fibers up to, and at times extending into, the lesion. This is consistent with the picture demonstrated by light microscopy. Thus, the lesion produced by the Nd: YAG laser and visualized by light microscopy is misleading in terms of size. Obviously, the functional size of the lesion is greater than what appears to be the anatomical size, though this regresses with time.

In an effort to explain the physiochemical changes noted, the thermal effects of each laser were examined. Using the same parameters previously described lesions were produced with either CO_2 or Nd: YAG laser at 25 watts at 0.5 second exposure at spot size 0.4 mm. Thus, lesions were of identical radiant exposure. Using a stereotactic procedure, microthermal couples were implanted at predetermined distances away from and deep to the lesion. Temperature changes were recorded over a one minute period following exposure. Each temperature reading is the average of 3 recordings. Each lesion was followed by a rapid raising temperature over 1.2 to 1.8 seconds which rapidly dropped over one minute to the baseline. With the CO_2 laser, (Fig. 3) the thermal changes were minimal, as close as .5 mm from the periphery and deep to the lesion. With the Nd: YAG laser (Fig. 4), on the other hand, the maximum heat was consistently greater 1 mm below the surface of the cortex; this remained a constant finding as far as 2 mm lateral to the lesion.

CONCLUSION

The use of Nd: YAG laser in neurosurgery is currently being investigated. Because the basic and clinical experience with CO_2 laser is so much more voluminous, this source is used as a standard against which other lasers are compared. Aside from the theoretical and practical advantages of YAG laser in effecting greater hemostasis and being transmittable through an optical cable,

144

the increased depth of destruction, both anatomic and physiologic, must be considered. On the other hand, as postulated by Beck and Ascher, the ability to produce heat effects deep to an intact structure offers certain engaging possibilities, particularly in the treatment of tumorous extension through venous sinus.

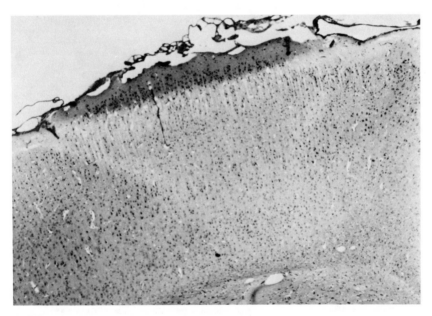

FIG. 1.   Immediate CO_2 Lesion

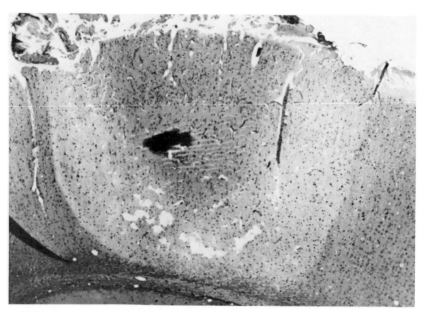

FIG. 2. Immediate Nd: YAG Lesion

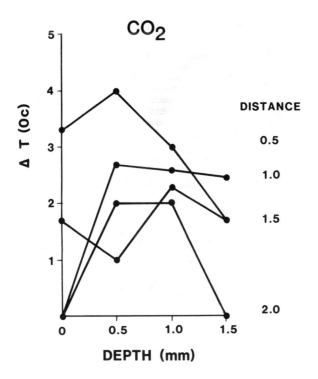

FIG. 3. Thermal Effects of the CO_2 Laser

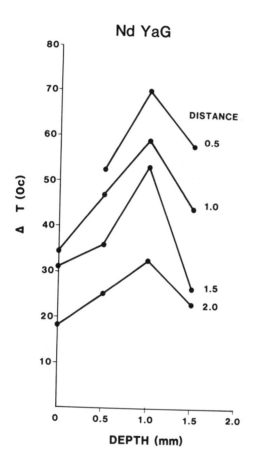

FIG. 4. Thermal Effect of the Nd: YAG Laser

148

REFERENCES

1.   J.C. Fisher, The Power Density of a Surgical Laser: Its Meaning and Measurement. Lasers in Surgery and Medicine 2, 301-315 (1983).

2.   M.L. Saunders, H.F. Young, D.P. Becker, et. al. The Use of the Laser in Surgery. Surg. Neurol. 14, 1-10 (1980).

3.   J.C. De La Torre, J.W. Surgon, Methodological Approach to Rapid and Sensitive Monoamine Histoflurosence Using a Modified Glyoxic Acid Technique; The SPC Method. Histochemistry 49, 81-93 (1976).

CHAPTER 17

THE Nd:YAG LASER IN OPHTHALMOLOGY - A REVIEW

Principal Author:
Paul R. Goth
American Hospital Supply Corporation
Irvine, California

THE Nd-YAG LASER IN OPHTHALMOLOGY

PAUL R. GOTH and STEPHEN M. FRY, Ph.D.
Medical Specialties Business
American Hospital Supply Corporation
2132 Michelson Drive
Irvine CA 92715

INTRODUCTION

Ophthalmologists have been pioneers in the application of laser technology to medicine.[1,2] The eye lends itself well to laser applications because its internal structures are easily accessible to most laser radiation through the clear cornea. The use of the Argon laser has revolutionized the treatment of diabetic retinopathy, retinal detachments and senile macular degeneration.

During the past year, there has been a second ophthalmic laser revolution — use of the ultra-short pulsed Neodymium:YAG laser for cutting intraocular tissue.[3,4] The Nd-YAG laser has been one of the hottest topics at both ophthalmic and technical conferences and many proposed uses are under investigation. In this chapter, we describe the laser systems currently being evaluated, how they work, what they can do in the eyes, and what safety aspects must be considered. We conclude with a discussion of probable future applications of both short-pulse and continuous wave Nd-YAG lasers in ophthalmology.

CLINICAL APPLICATIONS

Currently, all ophthalmic short-pulsed Nd-YAG lasers in the United States are being utilized under an investigational device exemption (IDE) from the Food and Drug Administration (FDA). In this section, we describe the primary application of the short-pulsed Nd-YAG laser in the eye and list some of the other uses for which investigations are being conducted.

The Nd-YAG laser application which has recently drawn attention in the ophthalmic community is the treatment of post-cataract opacifications. As people age, or if an eye is subjected to traumatic injury, a cataract may develop. A cataract is an opacification, or cloudiness, of the natural lens of the eye. The lens is enclosed and supported within a thin, clear capsule having anterior and posterior membranous surfaces. The most common treatment of a cataract is its surgical removal. There are several procedures by which a cataract may be removed and an increasingly common method is the extra-capsular cataract extraction (ECCE).

During an ECCE, the anterior surface of the capsule and the lens nucleus is removed leaving the posterior capsule intact. The refractive power of the removed natural lens is replaced using thick cataract spectacles, contact lenses or, more frequently, a small plastic intraocular lens (IOL). The IOL is positioned either in front of the iris or behind the iris just in front of the posterior capsule (Figure 1).

© 1983 by Elsevier Science Publishing Co., Inc.
Neodymium-YAG Laser in Medicine and Surgery, Joffe, Muckerheide, and Goldman, editors

Side View of Eye

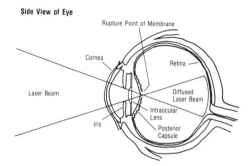

Figure 1. Structure of the eye showing location of posterior chamber IOL and laser beam focused on posterior capsule.

Over time 25% to 40% of post-ECCE patients develop opacifications of the posterior capsule which distort the visual image supplied to the retina. The patient experiences decreased vision, similar to looking through a piece of frosted glass or through a piece of wrinkled clear plastic film. Until recently, the remedy has been to surgically cut the membrane in a secondary procedure known as a posterior capsulotomy, or discission. The procedure is not a minor one, as it subjects the patient to the trauma of surgery and anesthesia again, and usually requires hospitalization and a short (two to three days) recuperative period.

With the advent of the short-pulsed ophthalmic Nd-YAG laser, posterior capsulotomy has become a five to ten minute non-invasive office procedure. The Nd-YAG laser beam passes through the cornea and creates an opening in the posterior capsule membrane that allows light to pass undistorted to the retina (Figure 1). The procedure requires no anesthesia, has an immediate effect on vision, and has no recuperative period.

Other applications under investigation include anterior capsulotomy prior to cataract surgery, cutting of anterior vitreous strands, synechotomy, iridotomy and iridectomy. As ophthalmologists gain more experience with the short-pulsed Nd-YAG laser, many other applications are being discovered.

LASER-TISSUE INTERACTIONS

Much work has shown that each laser wavelength interacts with each separate tissue type differently.[5,6,7,8,9,10] These effects can be attributed to different spectral absorption characteristics of tissue based on pigmentation, blood content, etc. For example, Argon laser light (488 - 514 nm) is absorbed three times more strongly than Nd-YAG energy (1064 nm) in the pigment epithelium of the eye (Figure 2). Tissue damage by laser radiation can occur through both the effects of linear and/or non-linear absorption of the energy.[11,12,13]

Linear absorption of laser radiation by an absorptive (opaque) tissue results in the conversion of light energy into heat. The photons contained in the beam of light are absorbed by the atoms and molecules of the target tissue increasing their

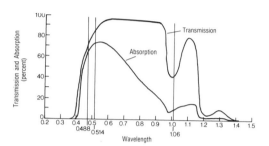

Figure 2. Transmission through ocular media and absorption in human retinal pigment epithelium.

vibrational energy. The temperature of the tissue increases through a transfer of the vibrational energy of the molecules to translational (kinetic) energy. If the temperature is raised sufficiently, protein denaturation and vaporization of the tissue can occur.

When a tissue is transparent to the wavelength of the incident light, no linear absorption occurs and no heating takes place. However, a focused high intensity laser beam, such as that in the ophthalmic Nd-YAG system, can cause disruption of tissue that is normally transparent through non-linear absorption.[3,11,12,14] This is achieved by obtaining optical power densities sufficient to cause electrostriction and dielectric breakdown. Optical breakdown (which appears as a small spark) occurs when electric fields induced by light energy are strong enough to strip electrons from their nuclei, causing ionization of the medium and the formation of a plasma. It is called "optical breakdown" since it is caused by light energy. Plasma, as used here, is a physics term referring to the ionized state of the medium, not a medical term referring to the fluid component of blood.

Optical breakdown results in the vaporization of a small volume of media and the creation of a transient shock wave which can disrupt adjacent tissues. The effect is similar to a controlled "microexplosion." It has been shown that these acoustic transients are spherical pressure waves with gradients as high as 900 mm Hg.[15] As the waves propagate, the pressure diminishes with the square of their radius.

Through the process of non-linear absorption resulting in optical breakdown, diaphanous transparent ocular tissues can be treated. If pigment, opacities, or structural interfaces are present, the optical breakdown threshold is decreased, probably through the addition of linear absorption effects.

To produce sufficiently strong electric fields for optical breakdown, a laser must produce a threshold irradiance of approximately 10^{10} W/cm^2. (Irradiance and power density are equivalent terms.)

$$\text{Irradiance} = \text{Energy} / \text{Time} / \text{Area}$$

A plasma "bubble" forms as soon as the instantaneous power density threshold is achieved. Further energy contained in the laser pulse tends to be absorbed

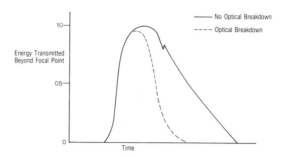

Figure 3.   Plasma shielding phenomenon in which tail of laser pulse is absorbed in plasma generated by optical breakdown.

or scattered in the plasma volume. Energy measurements taken along the beam propagation axis show that only 20% of incident energy passes through the region of optical breakdown[16] (Figure 3).

The fact that little energy is transmitted beyond the breakdown zone tends to protect subsequent structures (e.g., the retina) by reducing the incident irradiance. The ophthalmic literature has referred to this protection as "plasma shielding."[3,17,18,19] When working in the anterior segment of the eye, its importance in retinal safety seems to be secondary to other factors, as we shall discuss later. As deep posterior segment uses for the pulsed Nd-YAG are evaluated, plasma shielding may become more important.

Nd-YAG OPHTHALMIC LASERS

The threshold for optical breakdown requires a very high power density. Obtaining this threshold is the driving force behind the design of the short-pulsed Nd-YAG systems for ophthalmic applications. The ophthalmic Nd-YAG laser system is designed to ensure safety by minimizing both pulse energy and retinal irradiance. To minimize the pulse energy, the parameters available for manipulation are the pulsewidth of the laser and the spot size of the beam. Therefore, lasers with ultra-short pulsewidths are being used. The major characteristics of these lasers are:

- low energy output   (0.5 - 30 mJ)
- short pulse widths   (0.03 - 15 nsec)
- near IR wavelength   (1064 nm)
- small spot sizes   (.005 - .05 mm)
- high irradiances   (10^{10} W/cm^2)

Currently under investigation are two basic types of laser systems: Q-switched and mode-locked. There are significant differences in construction, as well as in the pulse and energy characteristics of these types of lasers. The Q-switched laser emits nanosecond (billionth of a second) pulses while the mode-locked laser emits picosecond (trillionth of a second) pulses.

In the development of pulsed Nd-YAG systems for clinical use, there have been significant discussions on the relative merits of mode-locking and Q-switching. We built the first prototype system which combined a mode-locked and a Q-switched laser into the same delivery optics. We have used the system to compare the two modalities side-by-side. Our results indicate that both systems are able to disrupt intraocular tissue, but we feel the Q-switched device has significant advantages.[20,21]

The main difference between a mode-locked laser and a Q-switched laser is the method of pulsing the output. Figures 4 and 5 compare typical pulse characteristics of a mode-locked laser to those of a Q-switched laser. A mode-locked laser utilizes an intra-cavity dye cell to emit seven to fifteen pulses, each typically 30 picoseconds long, approximately 4 nanoseconds apart. The pulse train contains between 3 to 6 mJ total energy depending upon the quality of the dye. The dye solution used to modulate the emission of energy degrades over time and must be replaced every two to eight weeks. The Q-switched laser utilizes a

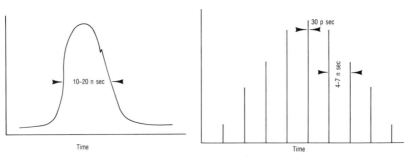

Figure 4. Typical pulse output of Q-switched Nd-YAG laser.

Figure 5. Typical pulse output of mode-locked Nd-YAG laser.

Pockel's Cell, an electro-optic "shutter," to emit a single 10 to 20 nsec pulse. The pulse energy is easily varied and typical ophthalmic systems can emit up to 30 mJ.

Whichever laser system is used, it is coupled to a standard slit lamp for delivery of the laser beam to the target area. Figure 6 is a photograph of a typical system. A slit lamp is a binocular microscope for examining the internal and external structures of the eye. It utilizes a focused slit of light for illumination, hence it's name. Visualization of the various structures of the eye is accomplished by moving the focal plane of the microscope in all three axes.

Coupling of the beam to the slit lamp is accomplished using mirrors, beam-splitters and, in some cases, articulating arms. Fiber optic cables are not used because the high power density of the laser radiation would damage the fiber input coupler.

The collimated beam emitted by the laser head is not useful for the safe generation of optical breakdown in the eye. With a low divergence beam there is no predictable site for breakdown to occur. In addition, the spot is very large and excessive pulse energies would be required to reach breakdown threshold. Finally, even if the energies were "low," they would most likely exceed the retinal irradiance damage threshold. All these problems are addressed using beam conditioning optics.

The beam conditioning optics expand the beam to a large diameter and then rapidly focus it. As the focus angle of the beam is increased (the f-number is decreased), the size of the focused spot decreases. A decreased spot size has two advantages: A lower energy requirement to achieve breakdown and a more sharply defined region in which breakdown can occur. Since breakdown occurs at a threshold power density, if the delivered energy is set to an appropriate level, the breakdown threshold is reached only at the focal point. It is important to note that, as the energy level is increased, the point at which breakdown occurs will move toward the focusing optics.[22]

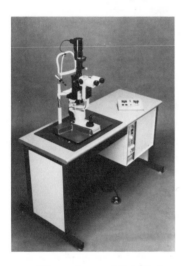

Figure 6. Q-Switched ophthalmic Nd-YAG laser sold under I D E by American Medical Optics, a Division of American Hospital Supply Corporation.

When a beam of light is focused, the light converges to a minimum spot size at the focal point and then diverges at approximately the same angle at which it was focused (Figure 7). As the distance from the focal point increases, the radiation is distributed over an exponentially larger area. This is the primary method by which the ophthalmic Nd-YAG laser systems reduce their corneal and retinal irradiances to safe non-damaging levels.

A visible beam aiming system is necessary to provide a means by which the invisible pulsed Nd-YAG beam may be applied to appropriate targets. The aiming beam is supplied by a low power Helium-Neon (HeNe) laser that emits a red (632.8 nm) beam which is focused at the same point as the Nd-YAG beam. Aiming is accomplished by looking through the microscope of the slit lamp and moving the slit lamp until the red spot appears on the target. As the slit lamp is moved, the target moves in and out of the focal plane causing the HeNe spot to grow and shrink. The Nd-YAG laser is fired when the red HeNe spot is its smallest diameter on the target tissue.

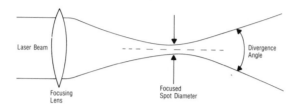

Figure 7. **Laser beam is first expanded, then focused to a beam waist. Diameter of waist is proportional to wavelength of light and inversely proportional to core angle.**

SAFETY CONSIDERATIONS

As with all laser systems, it is important to understand the possible risks associated with the use of the ophthalmic Nd-YAG laser. Since therapeutic lasers are designed to induce damage to pathologic structures, it follows that they are also capable of damaging healthy or normal structures as well. The ophthalmic Nd-YAG system is designed to disrupt tissues through the formation of optical breakdown in a three dimensionally defined region within the eye. To be safe in the use of this laser, it is important to know what undesirable effects are possible and how to minimize their occurrence.

For more than fifteen years, the military has studied and used pulsed Nd-YAG laser systems as target designators and rangefinders. Furthermore, the primary developers of the ophthalmic Nd-YAG therapy (Professors Aron-Rosa in Paris, France, and Fankhauser in Bern, Switzerland) have treated several thousand patients in their clinics. As a result, a large volume of data has been collected which gives significant insight into the effect of these lasers on the eye. A brief list of potential undesirable effects of the pulsed-YAG in the eye includes:

1. Tissue damage at the site of optical breakdown
2. Tissue damage remote from the site of optical breakdown
3. Tissue damage unrelated to optical breakdown
4. Damage to intraocular lenses (IOL's)

Tissue Damage at the Site of Optical Breakdown

The purpose of the ophthalmic Nd-YAG laser is to non-invasively cut intra-ocular tissue in a three-dimensionally defined area. The method by which this occurs is the formation of a mechanical shock wave which disrupts tissue at and near the site of optical breakdown. All available ophthalmic Nd-YAG systems provide an aiming system to properly position the beam within the eye.

In most instances, the physician desires tissue to be damaged at the point at which he aims the laser system. This requires the aiming beam to be in proper alignment with the therapeutic beam. If this is not the case, then tissue damage may occur in unexpected regions giving an undersirable result. Furthermore, if the Nd-YAG laser is accidentally fired when it is aimed at an inappropriate target, undesirable damage may also occur.

Another potential source for problems is that, as higher pulse energies are used, the region of optical breakdown moves toward the laser focusing optics. The shift occurs because breakdown is initiated at the first point at which the power density threshold is reached. With higher energies the threshold can be achieved earlier in the focused beam path. Van der Zypen[22] has reported a shift of up to 0.5 mm at 60 mJ energy levels. This offset can be minimized by using the lowest energy levels consistent with achieving optical breakdown and an adequate tissue effect.

In summary, to avoid accidental damage to the patient's eye, it is important that the operator regularly examine the positional relationship between the HeNe spot and the site of optical breakdown. Secondly, he should select this target carefully and fire only when he is sure he is accurately focused on it. And, finally, he should use the minimum amount of energy required to achieve an appropriate therapeutic result.

Tissue Damage Remote from the Site of Optical Breakdown

The effect of optical breakdown caused by a focused, short-pulsed Nd-YAG laser is similar to that of a microexplosion. A shock wave is formed which rapidly emanates from the focal point due to the rapid heating and phase change which can occur with optical breakdown.[23,24] It is this mechanical effect which is responsible for the disruption or cutting of intraocular membranes.[6,13,25] There is concern, however, that tissues remote from the site of optical breakdown may be damaged by these same forces.

Numerous investigators have found that tissue damage due to shock wave seems to be limited to the vicinity of the focal point of the laser beam. McNair[15] measured pressures as high as 900 mm Hg in the eyes of Rhesus monkeys subjected to optical breakdown with a xenon arc or a Ruby laser. He was unable to locate tissue damage, except in the region of the focal point.

Even though the pressure gradient is extremely high near the focal point, the wavefront rapidly propagates away from the site of breakdown. The wavefront propagation is analogous to the waves created by a rock thrown into a still pond. As the wavefront progresses, its pressure is reduced by the square of its distance from the focal point.

The initial wavefront is a sphere with a radius approximately equal to that of the focused beam spot. The ophthalmic Nd-YAG lasers produce focal spots with radii of .005 to .05 mm. With a simple calculation, it is apparent that the initial pressures have been reduced by a factor of 400 or more by the time the wavefront has expanded to 1 mm. This would suggest that the mechanical effects are very localized and present little danger to remote structures. Clinical experience in both Europe and the United States has shown no evidence of remote mechanical tissue damage.

Tissue Damage Unrelated to Optical Breakdown

One of the major concerns regarding the use of any laser is the capability of exposing the eye to sufficient energy to produce thermal burns. The retina, a structure comprised mainly of nerve tissue, warrants the most concern because, once injured, it is not capable of regenerating visual function.

Over the past 15 years extensive research has examined the effects of pulsed Nd-YAG laser radiation on the eye. When dealing with energy and power densities below the threshold required for optical breakdown, the tissue damage mechanisms are related to the absorption characteristics of the tissue and the power density of the laser pulse at the point it strikes the tissue.[10,11] The ophthalmic Nd-YAG lasers provide protection to non-target tissues by utilizing a wavelength which is only partially absorbed in critical tissues, by greatly reducing the power density of incident radiation through plasma absorption and by the use of sharply focusing optics which tend to disperse the beam over a large area beyond the focal region.

Figure 2 indicates the percent of light transmitted through the ocular media at various wavelengths. The percent transmission for 1064 nm in the preretinal media is 76% and only 23% is absorbed by the retina and choroid. Therefore, less than 24% of incident radiation is absorbed by the cornea and only 15% to 25% is absorbed by the retina.

A plasma bubble also absorbs and scatters a large amount of incident radiation. Studies have shown that as much as 80% to 90% of energy does not continue along the axis of propogation beyond the plasma region.[3,16,19] Part of that energy builds and maintains the plasma and the rest is scattered in all directions.[17,23] This effect reduces the energy incident on the retina but it is not the major protective factor since the occurrence of optical breakdown cannot be assured on every pulse.

Most non-target tissue protection is a result of the focusing optics dispersing the incident energy over large areas outside the focal region of the laser beam. The angle at which light is focused is called the cone angle. It is defined as the included angle delineated by two marginal rays, 180° apart, drawn from the focusing aperture to the focal point. Beyond the focal point, the beam diverges at the same angle. Currently available systems utilize a cone angle of 9° to 18° with 16° being most common.

When the beam is focused on the posterior capsule (5 mm behind the cornea and 15 mm in front of the retina), the spot size of the radiation that reaches the retina is in excess of 3 mm. Using the retinal damage threshold determined by Griess[26] (1064 nm, 16 nsec, 0.03 mm spot size) of 0.28×10^8 W/cm^2, the power density of the laser radiation drops below threshold levels 3.2 mm beyond the focal point. This implies that one may theoretically focus within 3.2 mm of the retina without causing threshold lesions. However, since the mechanisms for retinal damages are not fully understood, it is recommended that the minimum distance from the focal point to the retina be more than 5 mm.

As we have seen, the major protection for the cornea and retina is the dispersion of the beam over large areas through the use of sharply convergent focusing optics. The absorption and scatter of the laser radiation by the plasma bubble is a secondary protection in anterior segment procedures but may be more important as applications closer to the retina are investigated. To date, there has been no evidence of retinal damage in the application of pulsed Nd-YAG lasers in clinical ophthalmology.

Damage to Intraocular Lenses

One of the primary uses of the ophthalmic Nd-YAG laser is the opening of the posterior lens capsule following extra-capsular cataract extraction and intra-ocular lens implantation. Because the posterior capsule lies behind the IOL, it is necessary to deliver the energy through the IOL to the target tissue. Clearly, there is a potential for IOL damage if optical breakdown occurs in, or very near to, the IOL. If damage occurs, it appears as a small pit or surface cracking of the plastic or glass lens material. The extent of the damage depends upon the material composition of the IOL, the location of the breakdown with respect to the IOL, and the energy of the laser pulse.

Because the use of the short-pulsed Nd-YAG laser is new, in-depth studies of its effect on IOLs have not been published. Early evidence suggests that harder lenses may withstand laser radiation better than softer lenses. Glass lenses have higher laser damage thresholds than plastic lenses, but the threshold pit or crack is larger in the glass lenses.

Currently, it is recommended by Gentsler that energy levels below 5 mJ be used when irradiating tissue through an IOL. Furthermore, he recommends that multiple shots not be fired through the same spot in the IOL to reduce the potential for cumulative damage effects.

THE FUTURE OF THE Nd-YAG LASER IN OPHTHALMOLOGY

As the short-pulse Nd-YAG laser gains acceptance in performing non-invasive posterior capsulotomies, many investigators are now looking forward to increased use of this laser in the eye. The feasibility of cutting vitreous bands, strands and membranes has already been shown. There is ongoing research investigating the safety of applying the Nd-YAG laser (and resulting optical breakdown) closer to the retina. In addition, some investigators are attempting other anterior segment applications, including iridotomy/iridectomy, synechotomy, cyclodialysis and other potential treatments for glaucoma.

The short-pulse Nd-YAG lasers may also be enhanced through the use of "thermal mode" operation. Here, the Nd-YAG laser is operated with a longer pulse (neither Q-switched nor mode-locked) typically in the range of 5 to 10 mS. This allows the laser to heat tissue via the more conventional linear absorption process, causing coagulation, vaporization of tissue and thermal scars. For the Nd-YAG laser, linear absorption requires some pigmentation of the tissue; hemaglobin, melanin, and pigment epithelium all contribute to absorption of 1064 nm radiation. None of these have strong absorption peaks near the Nd-YAG wavelength, however, so the penetration depth of the Nd-YAG laser is relatively larger (of the order millimeters) than that of the CO_2 laser (tens of microns). This effect may be advantageous or disadvantageous depending on the intended application of the laser energy. The thermal mode Nd-YAG laser has been used in Europe,[22] but remains largely undeveloped at the present time.

Entirely new forms of laser energy can be created by doubling or tripling the frequency of the Nd-YAG laser through the non-linear effect of special crystals. The resulting 532 nm and 355 nm wavelengths are in the green and ultraviolet, respectively, and thus will interact with tissue quite differently from 1064 nm radiation. These non-linear effects, just as with optical breakdown, are power

160

dependent phenomena and require high peak powers (and generally short-pulse widths) for good efficiency. The effects of short-pulse green laser radiation on various structures of the eye have not been studied extensively, but could possibly yield some therapeutic benefit used in either non-linear (optical breakdown) or linear (heating) absorption modes. While longer pulse lengths would be required for true heating of tissue, one could also expect photochemical effects from the 532 nm and especially the 355 nm Nd-YAG wavelengths.

Finally, the discussion of Nd-YAG lasers would not be complete without touching on the continuous wave (CW) Nd-YAG laser. Laser surgery is maturing with the CO_2, Argon and Nd-YAG lasers playing major roles. Both CO_2 and Nd-YAG lasers can be used for heating tissue but, while the CO_2 laser is highly absorbed by water in cells causing vaporization and cautery of only small vessels, the Nd-YAG laser has a much greater penetration depth and can coagulate larger areas more effectively (the Argon ion laser can coagulate very effectively, due to the absorption of the green laser light by hemaglobin in red blood cells). The combination of Nd-YAG and CO_2 laser energy may prove to be useful for many surgical applications. While infrared-carrying fiber optics for CO_2 lasers exist but are mainly in the development stage, fibers for CW Nd-YAG laser radiation are readily available. Thus, ocular tumors or other tissue may in the future be removed through the use of Nd-YAG or a combination of Nd-YAG and CO_2 lasers introduced through optical fibers.

As with other applications of lasers, or other tools in the surgical armementarium for that matter, the use of the Nd-YAG laser in ophthalmology will depend on efficacy and safety, coupled with medical benefit and economic justification. The current use of the short pulse Nd-YAG laser for posterior capsulotomy appears to provide a safe, efficacious procedure which obviates the need for invasive surgery, recovery time, and patient discomfort. As the indications for use of the ophthalmic Nd-YAG laser increase, the economic application of this tool will become available to a wide cross section of ophthalmologists specializing in both the anterior and posterior segments. The second laser revolution in ophthalmology has begun; only the future will tell the eventual applications of this exciting new tool.

REFERENCES

1. Clayman HM, Lasers for ophthalmic surgery. J Am Intraocul Implant Soc 6:336-338, 1980.
2. Dixon JA, Surgical Applications of Lasers. Institute of Electrical and Electronics Engineers. Proceedings 70, 1982.
3. Aron-Rosa D, Aron JJ, Griesemann M, et al, Use of neodymium laser to open the posterior capsule after lens implant surgery. A preliminary report. J Am Intraocul Implant Soc 6:352-354, 1980.
4. Fankhauser FW, Roussel P, Steffen J, et al, Clinical studies on the efficiency of high power laser radiation upon some structures of the anterior segment of the eye. Int Ophthal 3:129-139, 1981.
5. Beatrice ES, Randolph DI, Zwick H, et al, Laser Hazards: Biomedical Threshold Level Investigations. Mil. Med 141(11):889-892, 1977.
6. Goldman A, Ham W, Mueller HA, Ocular damage thresholds and mechanisms for ultrashort pulses of both visible and infrared laser radiation in the rhesus monkey. Exp Eye Res 24:45-56, 1977.
7. Klein E, et al, Interaction of Laser Radiation with Biologic Systems I-III. Fed Proc 24:S35, S104, S143, 1965.

8. Geeraets WJ, Berry R, Ocular spectral characteristics as related to hazards from lasers and other light sources. Am J Ophthalmol 66:15-20, 1968.
9. Ham WT, Williams RC, Mueller HA, et al, Effects of laser radiation on the mammalian eye. Trans NY Acad Sci 28 (Ser 11):517-526, 1966.
10. Sliney D, Wolbarsht M, Safety with lasers and other optical sources. New York, Plenum Press, 1980.
11. Cleary SF, Laser pulses and the generation of acoustic transients in biological material, in Wolbarsht ML (ed): Laser Applications in Medicine and Biology Vol 3. New York, Plenus Press, 1977, pp. 175-219.
12. Cleary SF, Hamrick PE, Laser-induced acoustic transients in the mammalian eye. J Acoust Soc Amer 46:1037-1044, 1969.
13. Goldman AL, Ham WT, Mueller HA, Mechanisms of retinal damage resulting from the exposure of rhesus monkeys to ultrashort laser pulses. Exp Eye Res 21:457-469, 1975.
14. Griessman JC, et al, Thermal wave propagation and shock formation in ultrashort optical breakdown. J Appl Physiol 50:3915-3920, 1979.
15. McNair J, Franufelder FT, Wilson RS, et al, Acute pressure changes and possible secondary tissue changes due to laser or xenon photocoagulation. Am J Ophthalmol 77:13-18, 1974.
16. Steinert R, Puliafito C, Nd-YAG Laser Symposium, Ohio State University, September 1982.
17. Shkarofsky IP, Review of Gas-Breakdown Phenomena Induced by High-Power Lasers-I. RCA Review 35:48-77, 1974.
18. Aron-Rosa D, 'Cold' laser for eye microsurgery described by French Ophthalmologist. Ophthalomology Times 7(8), June 15, 1982
19. Aron-Rosa D, Griesseman J, Aron J, Use of a pulsed neodymium Nd-YAG laser (picosecond) to open the posterior capsule in traumatic cataract: A preliminary report. Ophthalmic Surg 12:494-499, 1981.
20. Keates R, "Interview: Neodymium—YAG Lasers Cut Clear Membranes." Ophthalmology Times 7(6), June 1, 1982.
21. Keates R, Fry S, Link W, Ophthalmic Nd-YAG Lasers Slack, New Jersey, 1983.
22. Van der Zypen E, Bebie H, Frankhauser F, Morphological studies about the efficiency of laser beams upon the structures of the angle of the anterior chamber. Int Ophthalmol 1:109-122, 1979.
23. Bell CE, Lanott JA, Laser-Induced High-Pressure Shock Waves in Water. Applied Physics Letters 10(2):46-48, 1967.
24. Saunders ML, et al, The Use of the Laser in Neurological Surgery. Surg Neurol 14:1-10, 1980.
25. Ham WT, Mueller HA, Goldman A, Ocular hazard from picosecond pulses of Nd-YAG laser radiation. Science 185:362, 1974.
26. Griess GA, Blankenstein MF, Ocular damage from multiple pulse laser exposures. Health Phys 39:921-927, 1980.

ADDITIONAL BIBLIOGRAPHY

Cain CP, et al, Measured and Predicted Laser-induced Temperature Rises in the Rabbit Fundus. Invest Ophthalmol 13:60, 1974.
Cleary SF, Laser-induced Temperature Transients. Va J Sci 19:205, 1968.
Fine S, Klein E, Nowak W, et al, Interaction of laser radiation with biologic systems. 1. Studies on interaction with tissues. Fed Proc Fed Amer Soc Exp Biol 24 (pt 3):35-47, 1965.
Fankhauser FW, "Swiss Scientist Disputes French laser Statements." Ophthalmology Times 7(9), June 15, 1982.
Krasnov MM, Laser Phakopuncture in the treatment of soft cataracts. Br J Ophthalmol 59:96-98, 1975.
Marshall J, Thermal and mechanical mechanisms in laser damager to the retina. Invest Ophthalmol Vis Sci 9:97-115, 1970.

Van der Zypen E, Frankauser F, Bebie H, On the effects of different laser energy sources upon the iris of the pigmented and the albino rabbit. Int Ophthal 1:30-48, 1978.

Van der Zypen E, Frankhauser F, Bebie H, et al, Changes in the ultrastructure of the iris after irradiation with intense light. Adv Ophthalmol 39:59-180, 1979.

Van der Zypen E, Frankhauser F, The ultrastructural features of laser trabeculo-puncture and cyclodialysis. Ophthalmologica 179:189-200, 1979.

CHAPTER 18

THE Nd:YAG LASER IN OPHTHALMOLOGY

Robert H. Osher, M.D.
Cincinnati Eye Institute
Cincinnati, Ohio

THE NEODYMIUM - YAG LASER IN OPHTHALMOLOGY

Robert H. Osher, M.D., Cincinnati Eye Institute, Cincinnati, Ohio

The ophthalmic Neodymium-YAG laser, since its immigration into the United States in 1982, has created tremendous interest in noninvasive intraocular surgery. Two European physicians, Daniele Aron-Rosa, M.D. from France and Franz Fankhauser, M.D. from Switzerland have independently developed and explored the clinical potential of this laser in eye surgery. Dr. Aron-Rosa's original laser was provided by the arms industry, while Dr. Fankhauser's laser was borrowed from the microprocessing industry. Although ophthalmology was among the first specialties to demonstrate clinical application of thermal lasers, all American ophthalmologists are indebted to these individuals for introducing the "cold cutting" laser. The majority of our current information has originated from our European colleagues.

The unique characteristic of the Nd:YAG irradiation which has been responsible for the unprecedented popularity within ophthalmology, is the capability to selectively cut non-pigmented tissue within the eye. By either utilizing a Q-switched nanosecond (billionth of a second) pulse or mode-locked picosecond (trillionth of a second) pulse, an extremely high energy density is produced which tears atoms apart. The electrons that are ripped off the atom form a plasma shield which provides a relative screen of laser energy from further penetrating the eye. This plasma shield affords relative protection to the deeper structures, most importantly, the retina. As the electrons return to their atoms, a spark much like a miniature lightening bolt is created and a centrifugal shock wave is propagated which mechanically disrupts and vaporizes the target tissue. Since the wavelength of 1064 nm is invisible, a coaxial helium neon laser is used for aiming the YAG beam.

The YAG laser has the greatest potential application in cataract surgery, although its role in corneal, glaucoma, and vitreoretinal surgery is enthusiastically being explored. To appreciate the usefulness to the cataract surgeon, one must understand the meaning and management of the cataract.

The crystalline lens is the transparent focussing device inside the eye which is located behind the iris and pupil and is suspended in place by fine linear web-like structures known as the zonules (Figure 1). When an object is at different distances from the eye, the lens must change shape to maintain perfect focus of the image onto the retina (the natural lens is analogous to the lens of a camera and the retina is similar to the film). For reasons we do not understand, age and other factors may cause the lens to lose its clarity and opacification develops. This clouding of the lens is defined as a cataract.

When the vision resulting from the cataract is no longer acceptable for the patient to fulfill his visual needs and to enjoy the quality of his life, then elective cataract surgery is indicated. Over 600,000 operations are performed annually and half of these are combined with the implantation of an intraocular lens.

Traditionally, the cataract was removed by opening the eye 180° and placing a freezing probe upon the lens surface after an enzyme was used to "dissolve" the supporting zonules. The probe, when activated, would create an iceball that would adhere to the lens and the entire cataract could be removed as the surgeon withdrew the probe (Figure 2). This procedure was termed "intracapsular" and

© 1983 by Elsevier Science Publishing Co., Inc.

Neodymium-YAG Laser in Medicine and Surgery, Joffe, Muckerheide, and Goldman, editors

165

the results were generally excellent.

With the advent of new techniques such as "phacoemulsification", incisions that were one sixth of the previous wound (3 mm.) would permit an ultrasonic probe to enter the eye and the cataract could be broken into tiny fragments which were then removed through the small opening (Figure 3). Additional wound strength and rapid visual rehabilitation were among the advantages, yet more importantly these "extracapsular" methods preserved the back surface of the lens known as the posterior capsule, which was polished and left intact. The additional stability to the back of the eye offered a significant reduction in the dreaded complications of retinal swelling (cystoid macular edema) and retinal detachment following cataract surgery.

Furthermore, new intraocular lenses were designed to occupy the same location as the human lens. The implant was inserted behind the iris where it was supported by the posterior capsule (Figure 4). These intraocular lenses offered optimal physiologic vision, added additional stability to the vital structures in the back of the eye, allowed the pupil to be dilated, appear cosmetically indetectable, and were remotely situated from the other delicate structures of the eye.

Therefore, the advantage of the "extracapsular" techniques was the protection afforded by the preserved posterior capsule. Yet the posterior capsule also was the source of a new problem since a significant percentage of patients (approximately 30%) would develop clouding of these capsules years following surgery and the vision would decrease (Figure 5). Many of these patients required another operation to open the membrane, incurring the expense and undergoing the risk (hemorrhage, infection, retinal disease) of disturbing the eye again. Some surgeons concluded that the posterior capsule could be opened at the time of surgery in order to avoid possible re-operation in the future. Yet few would argue against the maximum safety afforded by leaving the posterior capsule intact, especially in patients at high risk for complications following surgery.

The ability to leave the capsule intact at surgery and open it with the laser at a later time if necessary without requiring another operation is probably the most helpful application of the YAG laser today (Figure 6). In most instances, a small number of shots are required to produce an opening in the posterior capsule coinciding with the visual axis. All of the initial reports from the Eruopeans who have performed 8,000 cases and from a smaller number in the United States indicate that this is a safe and effective procedure, with immediate restoration of vision.

While some investigators are studying the effect of the laser on an intraocular lens, others are exploring the potential of the YAG laser to perform different parts of the cataract operation. Although an anterior capsulotomy can be performed with the laser, limited reports of increased intraocular pressure and inflammation have led to a cautious posture taken by the surgical community. Furthermore, once the laser anterior capsulotomy is performed, the surgeon is obligated to proceed with the operation so that cataract surgery loses its electivity.

Other indications for the YAG laser include:

(1) Sutures can be cut that have been used inside the eye for repairing the iris or stabilizing an intraocular lens. External sutures that have been used for closure of the surgical wound and are associated with either

irritation or astigmatism may also be exploded.

(2) The prolene loops of an intraocular lens may be cut if an implant requires removal.

(3) Adhesions around the pupil or inflammatory membranes following cataract surgery may be eliminated.

(4) An updrawn pupil may be enlarged by extending the opening into the optical zone, although a thermal laser with coagulation capability is probably preferable.

(5) An intraocular cyst may be eradicated.

(6) A peripheral iridectomy may be created, although again, there is an overlapping role with the thermal lasers.

(7) Peripheral anterior synechiae may be eliminated to prevent further zippering of the angle.

(8) A surgical fistula may be re-opened following glaucoma surgery.

(9) A graded trabeculectomy can be performed where the filtration can be increased by modifying the scleral flap sutures on the flap itself.

(10) Immediate lowering of the intraocular pressure following cataract surgery can be achieved by cutting sutures and creating a filtering bleb.

(11) Non-invasive goniotomy may be performed in congential glaucoma.

(12) Destruction of surface corneal ulcers or stromal microabscesses is possible.

(13) Vitreous bands may be severed especially when associated with traction induced cystoid macular edema, retinal detachment, or retinal tear formation.

(14) Avascular vitreous opacities and troublesome floaters may be obliterated.

Conclusion

The Nd:YAG laser has afforded the ophthalmologist an entirely new concept of intraocular surgery. The potential is endless. and we have not yet scratched the surface of therapeutic indications. The YAG laser is in its infancy much like the first generation CAT scanners. Yet we can be certain that tremendous advances in technology and knowledge will be forthcoming and our patients will reap the benefits.

167

NATURAL LENS

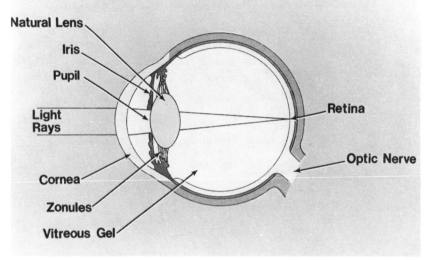

Figure 1.

CATARACT EXTRACTION
INTRACAPSULAR TECHNIQUE

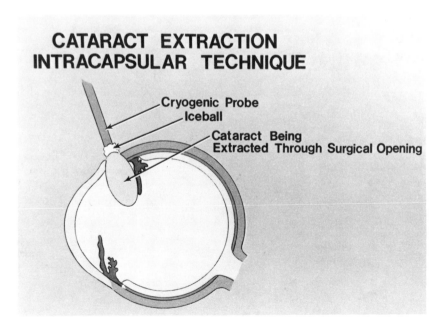

Figure 2.

168

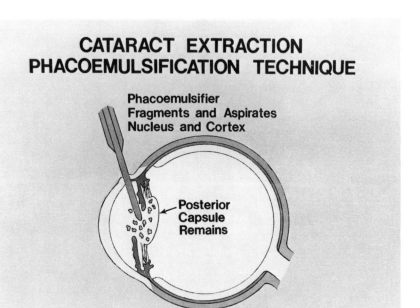

CATARACT EXTRACTION
PHACOEMULSIFICATION TECHNIQUE

Phacoemulsifier
Fragments and Aspirates
Nucleus and Cortex

Posterior
Capsule
Remains

Figure 3.

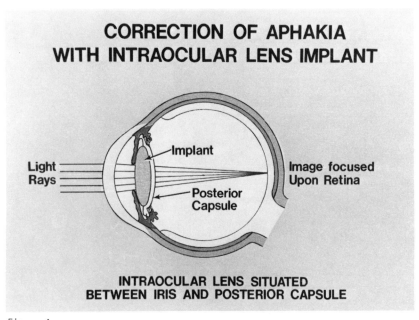

CORRECTION OF APHAKIA
WITH INTRAOCULAR LENS IMPLANT

Implant

Light
Rays

Image focused
Upon Retina

Posterior
Capsule

INTRAOCULAR LENS SITUATED
BETWEEN IRIS AND POSTERIOR CAPSULE

Figure 4.

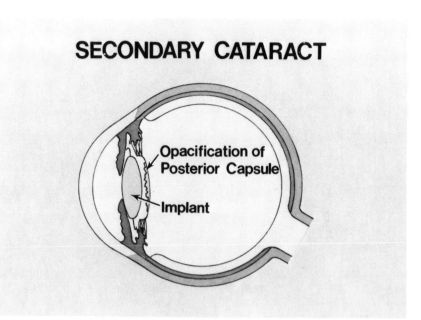

Figure 5.

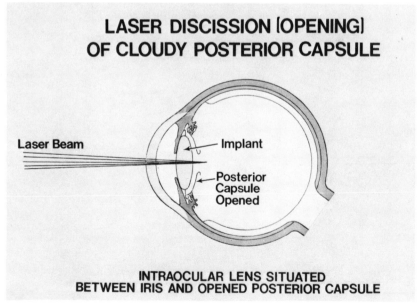

Figure 6.

CHAPTER 19

THE Nd:YAG LASER IN GYNECOLOGY

Helmut F. Schellhas, M.D.
Department of Obstetrics and Gynecology
Univ. of Cincinnati Medical Center
and
The Laser Laboratory
The Jewish Hospital
Cincinnati, Ohio

172

THE NEODYMIUM-YAG LASER IN GYNECOLOGY

H. F. SCHELLHAS, M.D.
Department of Obstetrics and Gynecology, University of Cincinnati Medical Center,
231 Bethesda Avenue, Cincinnati, Ohio 45267, and The Laser Laboratory of The
Jewish Hospital of Cincinnati, 3200 Burnet Avenue, Cincinnati, Ohio 45229

CONTROL OF HEMORRHAGE AND DESTRUCTION OF MALIGNANT TUMORS

The neodymium YAG (Nd-YAG) laser beam has been used for hemostatic purposes mainly in the field of gastro-enterology. For the control of bleeding vessels the lowest possible power is utilized with an effort to keep ensuing tissue necrosis at a minimum. The diameter of the incident beam has therefore been focused to a very small size for the precise coagulation of small bleeding vessels in otherwise normal tissue. In oncology a controlled large volume tissue coagulation is desired and for this reason a high laser power output is used. Since tumor volumes are relatively expansive a large beam size is required in oncology. Tumor tissue, on the other hand, favors Nd-YAG laser beam absorption since it causes less back scattering than healthy tissue [1].

The scattering effect around the incident ND-YAG laser beam within the tissue heats up a large tissue volume and causes tissue coagulation without its removal. Tissue vaporization can be achieved by further heat generation of the coagulated and desiccated tissue with high energy densities and an added time factor. Large incisions with wide marginal necrotic tissue zones can be made with absolute hemostasis in the lower female genital tract.

Tumor destruction can be achieved in experimental animals in 4 to 5 mm tumors using 5 to 7 pulses of 40 W and 2 seconds duration [2]. Small tumors of the penis were destroyed by Hofstetter and Frank with a power output of 40 W and total energy of 1600 to 2400 Ws [3].

In gynecologic oncology the Nd-YAG laser has been used effectively to destroy tumor tissue in clinical situations in which tumors have recurred after previous radiation therapy in which the localization of the tumor does not allow surgical resection or where surgery is contraindicated because of severe medical problems or advanced age. Hemorrhage caused by recurrent tumor can be controlled by tissue coagulation. The author has utilized the Nd-YAG laser in the palliative treatment of patients with hemorrhaging tumors of the cervix and ovary metastatic to the vagina [4]. The laser beam was delivered by means of a handpiece using the model 8000 of the Molectron Corporation. The power of 40 to 100 W was used with the maximal pulse selection of 9.9 seconds and multiple pulse irradiation. The total energy ranged between 630 and 12,100 Ws.

Compared with other established treatment methods the Nd-YAG laser has the advantage of both, causing tumor destruction and hemostasis. The carbon dioxide laser can provide tumor destruction as long as hemorrhage is absent. A covering layer of blood will absorb the carbon dioxide laser beam and render it ineffective. Cryosurgery can freeze a bleeding tumor surface but provides only very superficial tumor destruction. A frozen tumor surface can be vaporized with the carbon dioxide laser to a tissue depth containing intact blood vessels and repeat freezing is required to allow further effective tissue vaporization [5]. Finally, obliteration of the internal iliac arteries for hemorrhaging vascular tumors by transcatheteral injection of gel foam particles and small steel spirals in our experience is the most effective and the longest lasting hemostatic procedure. The disadvantage is, however, that systemic chemotherapy will not reach the tumor cells when the blood vessels are obstructed. Laser photo-irradiation of hematoporphyrin fluorescent tumors by means of a rhodamine-B-dye laser is another alternative to Nd-YAG laser tissue coagulation of superficially invasive malignancies of the lower female genital tract [5] or extended carcinoma in situ.

The presently commercially available Nd-YAG lasers were mainly developed for the treatment of severe bleeding in gastro-enterology. Therefore the Nd-YAG lasers presently marketed are not ideally suited for use in oncology. The gynecologic oncologist will in most instances use an institutional Nd-YAG laser mainly acquired for use in gastro-enterology and neurosurgery. For clinical applications as described in this chapter we will find this laser system adequate though somewhat limited. Large cancer institutions should consider to have powerful Nd-YAG lasers custom built for the use of large spot sizes and high energy densities [7].

ENDOMETRIAL ABLATION THROUGH A HYSTEROSCOPE

Gynecologists have established a variety of endoscopic procedures for diagnostic and therapeutic purposes such as colposcopy, laparoscopy and hysteroscopy. Since the Nd-YAG laser beam can be delivered through a flexible quartz fiberoptic system and the penetration depth of the beam is predictable and controllable the Nd-YAG laser beam lends itself to therapeutic endoscopic application in gynecology.

Goldrath, Fuller and Segal have developed a method to destroy endometrium with the Nd-YAG laser beam through a hysteroscope [8]. The clinical indication was excessive and disabling uterine bleeding in patients not desirous of a hysterectomy. The surgical procedure is done under general or spinal anesthesia. The fallopian tubes are closed laparoscopically with a Yoon ring. The endometrial cavity is inspected by a hysteroscope and irrigated with 5% dextrose in 0.9% sodium chloride. Not more than 2.5 to 3 liters are used. The irrigation fluid is allowed to flow freely around the hysteroscope. A fiberoptic light guide is inserted through the operating channel of the hysteroscope. The operator's eyes are protected through a special filter or goggles. The surgeon uses a power output of 55 to 60 W and moves the hysteroscope continuously to cover the entire surface of the endometrial cavity with the fiberoptic tip in close approximation to the surface. The length of the uterine cervix is marked on the hysteroscope for identification and avoidance of treatment since coagulation of the high endocervix might induce hemorrhage. The procedure takes 30 to 40 minutes to perform. The clinical results were found to be excellent with the first group of 21 patients evaluated. Sero-sanguinous discharge was experienced up to 3 weeks. Hysterograms 3 to 6 months postoperatively showed marked scarring and deformity of the uterine cavity which often was found very contracted. Biopsies of the endometrial surface showed small amounts of endometrial glands which clinically was inconsequential. There was no inflammatory reaction other than foreign body giant cells surrounding carbon particles. A hysterectomy specimen 10 months after laser treatment showed the endometrial cavity lined by a simple mullerian type epithelium adjacent to the normal appearing myometrium. No inflammation was present and few carbon particles found.

This coagulation method of the endometrium by means of the Nd-YAG laser is an alternative to hysterectomy for functional endometrial bleeding. Goldrath reports also encouraging results in patients treated for submucous leiomyomas. The advantage to hysterectomy is obviously a minor surgical procedure with less morbidity and shorter hospitalization. Cost effectiveness of the laser procedure is another important consideration.

Nd-YAG LASER HAZARDS

The "laser gynecologist" trained in the use of the popular carbon dioxide laser has to be well familiar with the much more hazardous Nd-YAG laser. The basic physics of the Nd-YAG laser, the properties of the laser beam and the biologic effects are very different from the carbon dioxide laser. Nd-YAG laser surgical standards and safety measures need to be established. Every person directly or indirectly involved in Nd-YAG laser surgery also requires adequate knowledge of the laser hazards. Hospital safety precautions should provide adequate isolation of the operating room against the possibility of straying beams outside through an uncovered window or open door. Successful laser surgery can only be performed by a surgeon skilled in the use of the laser instrument.

REFERENCES

1. Buchholz J, Haverkampt K, Meyer HJ, Grotelueschen B, Borchers L: Scattering effects in laser surgery. in Kaplan I (editor): Laser Surgery II, Jerusalem Academic Press, Jerusalem, 1978
2. Staehler G, McCord RC, Hofstetter A and Keiditsche E: Nd-YAG laser irradiation of the normal and tumorous bladder wall. in Kaplan I (editor), Laser Surgery II, Jerusalem Academic Press, Jerusalem, 1978
3. Hofstetter H, and Frank F: The Neodymium-YAG laser in urology. Basle: Editiones Roche, 1980
4. Schellhas HF and Weppelmann B: The Neodymium-YAG laser in the treatment of gynecologic malignancies. Laser in Surgery and Medicine, Submitted
5. Schellhas HF: Cryogens and carbon dioxide laser in cyclic combination for volume reduction of vascular tumors in Kaplan I (editor): Laser Surgery III, Part I, OT-PAS, Tel Aviv, 1979
6. Ward BG, Forbes AJ, Cowled PA, et al: The treatment of vaginal recurrences of gynecologic malignancy with phototherapy following hematoporphyrin derivative pretreatment. Am J Obstet Gynecol 142,356-357, 1982
7. Muckerheide MC, St. Mary's Hospital, Milwaukee, Wisc. Personal Communication
8. Goldrath MH, Fuller A and Segal S: Laser photovaporization of the endometrium for the treatment of menorrhagia. Am J Obstet Gynecol 140:14-19, 1981

CHAPTER 20

FIRST EXPERIENCES WITH THE Nd:YAG LASER IN DERMATOLOGY

Principal Author:

M. Landthaler, M.D.
Department of Dermatology
University of Munich
Munich, Germany

176

FIRST EXPERIENCES WITH THE Nd:YAG LASER IN DERMATOLOGY

M. Landthaler[1], R. Brunner[1], D. Haina[2], F. Frank[3], W. Waidelich[2,4]
and O. Braun-Falco[1]

1) Department of Dermatology, University of Munich
   (Head Professor Dr. H.C. O. Braun-Falco)

2) Gesellschaft fur Strahlen- und Umweltforschung m.b.H.,

3) MBB-AT G.m.b.H., Munich

4) Institute for Medical Optics, University of Munich
   (Head Prof. Dr. W. Waidelich)

The argon laser is well established in plastic surgery and dermatology for treatment of vascular lesions like port wine stains, teleangiectases, and venous lakes due to its high absorption of the blue and green light bands.[1,2]

The CO_2 laser is widely used for removal of tattoos and virus papillomas,[2] and for excisions of skin tumors.[3,4,5]

Although the Nd:YAG laser is successfully employed in urology for treatment of benign and malignant tumors of the external genitalia,[6,7] there are only a few reports about the use of this laser for treatment of skin lesions.[8,9,10]

Since only little is known about depth of coagulation caused by Nd:YAG laser irradiation of human skin, experimental investigations were performed to elucidate this problem.

EXPERIMENTAL INVESTIGATIONS

Material and methods: For experiments and treatment of patients a 100 watt Nd:YAG laser (medilas, MBB-AT, Munich) was used. The laser beam was transmitted by a quartz fiber optic to a handpiece. By means of two lenses in this handpiece the laser beam was focused to a 2 mm spot size on skin, if distance between the handpiece and skin was 50 mm.

Uninvolved skin of full thickness with subcutaneous fat, which was excised in patients with malignant melanomas on the trunk, was employed. The skin was lasered with single pulses. Exposure time was 1,3 and 10 seconds per pulse. Laser power at the end of the focusing handpiece varied from 18 to 40 watts.

In one volunteer patient a written consent was obtained after a detailed description of the procedure. Thus, depth of coagulation could be investigated in vivo. Two single laser pulses were given in local anesthesia using mepivacain-HCl (Scandicain) on the skin of the chest. Spot size was 2 mm. Laser power at the end of the focusing handpiece was 50 watts, and exposure time 1 and 3 seconds respectively. During lasering the surface was chilled with a saline solution. The two skin lesions were excised after 48 hours in local anesthesia.

The skin of in vitro and in vivo experiments was processed in a routine histological fashion and stained by hemalam and eosin. Size and configuration of coagulation necrosis was measured by means of a calibrated measuring ocular.

Results: The in vitro experiments demonstrated dependence of depth of coagulation from laser power and exposure time. It extended from 0.4 to 4.1 mm (Fig. 1).

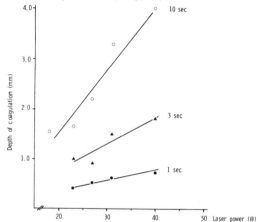

Fig. 1. Depth of coagulation caused by Nd:YAG laser irradiation of excised human skin in vitro.

Applying an exposure time of 1 sec. configuration of coagulation necrosis was nearly hemispheric, with longer exposure times more cylindric.

Overlying epidermis was coagulated also and separated from dermis by a subepidermal blister. The breadth of epidermal alteration exceeded that of the dermis. The ratio of epidermal to dermal alteration ranged between 1.1:1 and 1.4:1.

Depth of coagulation 48 hours after lasering measured 2.2 mm (1s, 50w) and 3.2 mm (3s, 50w) respectively.

Discussion: The in vitro experiment demonstrated that depth of coagulation in human skin was well assessable by variation of exposure time and power of the Nd:YAG laser beam. Coagulation depth in vivo was greater than in vitro, using excised human skin. This can be explained by the fact that after thermal injuries progressive tissue death continues for hours. The definitive depth of coagulation therefore could not be found immediately after the laser pulse. Additionally, chilling the surface increased depth of coagulation.[11] The attainable coagulation depth with the Nd:YAG laser exceeds by far that of the argon laser, which coagulates only superficially up to a maximum depth of 0.8 to 1.0 mm[12,13] (own unpublished data).

Clinical Applications

After having done these experimental investigations to elucidate coagulation depth of the Nd:YAG laser patients afflicted with various skin lesions were treated with this laser. All treatments were performed under local anesthesia, using mepivacain-HCl (Scandicain).

Skin tumors: In four patients a total of 10 nodular basal cell carcinomas were treated, employing a spot size of 2 mm, a laser power of 40 watts, and an exposure time between 1 and 3 seconds. The tumors were completely covered with laser pulses. A biopsy taken in one patient 48 hours after laser treatment demonstrated sufficient and deep coagulation of the tumor (Fig.2). Healing of the laser treated area lasted four to six weeks. Biopsies after complete healing revealed a thin epidermis and fibrosis of dermis, but no tumor cells.

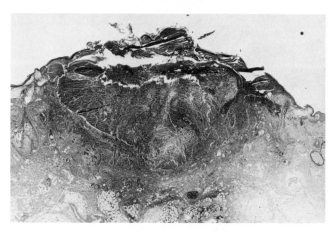

Fig. 2. Histology of basal cell carcinoma 48 hours past laser therapy, H and E staining, x 20.

Multiple superficial basal cell carcinomas could be removed by means of the Nd:YAG laser (10 to 20 w, 1.0 s).

Furthermore, patients suffering from bowenoid papulosis, oral florid papillomatosis, M. Bowen, solar keratosis and multiple skin metastases of malignant melanoma were treated.

Port wine stains: In 9 patients afflicted with extensive deep purple port wine stains with nodular surface test treatments were performed mainly in the retroauricular regions. Up to 10 Nd:YAG laser pulses (0.5 s, 20w) were set in alternative rows and stripes. Immediately after treatment the skin was whitish discolored, but the coagulation of skin was clinically not as regular as after argon laser pulses (Fig. 3a). Within 2 to 4 days the treated areas were covered by a scab, which separated after 2 to 3 weeks. Twelve weeks after treatment there was a marked lightening of the laser treated skin (Fig. 3b). But a few of the Nd:YAG lasered rows were slightly depressed, indicating some scar formation.

Histologically there was necrosis of the epidermis and dermis immediately after laser treatment. Dilated vessels down to a depth of 2 mm were filled with coagulated erythrocytes. After 6 days there was initial restoration of the epidermis. The dermis was coagulated to a depth of 1.5 mm and dilated vessels were filled with agglutination thrombi. In dermal layers beyond 1.5 mm fibroblasts and capillary blood vessels grew into the thrombi (Fig. 4).

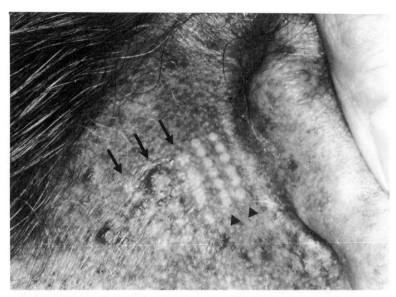

Fig. 3a. Argon (▲) and Nd:YAG (⬆) lasered rows immediately after irradiation

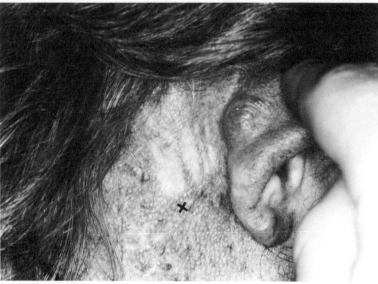

Fig. 3b. Marked lightening 12 weeks past therapy. Confluence of two Nd:YAG lasered rows (x) led to a broad blanching.

Later on deep and also superficial vessels were replaced by granulation tissue and after 2 to 4 weeks by newly formed fibrous tissue rich of fibroblasts.

In a 39 year old male patient afflicted with an extensive port wine stain of the face and labial hypertrophy (Fig. 5a) the lower lip was treated twice in a 6 weeks interval with the Nd:YAG laser. About 170 single pulses (20 w, 0.5 s) were given and a marked reduction in size of the lower lip could be obtained (Fig. 5b).

Discussion: Although our experiments in the treatment of skin tumors with the Nd:YAG laser are still limited and we don't yet have a sufficient follow-up of patients, our first clinical and histological findings are promising. Nd:YAG laser treatment may become an enrichment in therapy of skin tumors, since it can be performed easily and quickly with only local anesthesia on an out patient basis with little risk of bleeding and infection. It can be considered as certain that after gaining sufficient experience and clinical evidence in the treatment of benign and semimalignant tumors Nd:YAG laser irradiation will find definite indications also in the therapy of malignant tumors of the skin.

Additionally, the Nd:YAG laser may enrich treatment modalities for port wine stains. While in port wine stains of younger patients the number of dilated vessels is maximal in the immediate subepidermal area, it is well known that in older patients ectatic vessels can be found in deep layers of the skin. These deeper located vessels cannot be reached by the argon laser irradiation. In contrast our first clinical and histological examinations with the Nd:YAG laser demonstrated that even these deeply located vessels could be reached. This is important for treatment of deep purple port wine stains with nodular surface and labial hypertrophy. At the moment investigations are carried out to determine optimal parameters of irradiation and to improve treatment techniques including chilling of the surface, because in our experience Nd:YAG laser therapy is still burdened with a higher risk of scar formation compared to argon laser therapy.

This way, though, we believe that the Nd:YAG laser will establish in the treatment of special, deeply located vascular skin lesions.

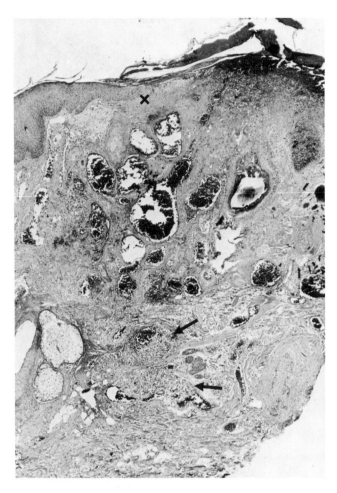

Fig. 4. Histology of a Nd:YAG laser treated port wine stain 6 days past treatment. Initial restoration of epidermis (x). Superficial ectatic vessels filled with coagulated erythrocytes. Vessels beyond 1.5 mm replaced by granulation tissue (↑). H&e-staining, x40.

182

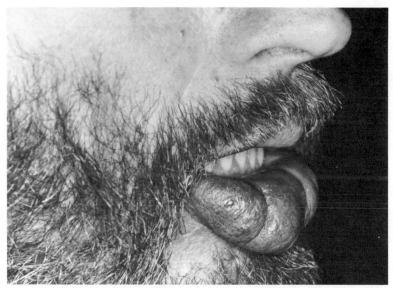

Fig. 5a. Labial hypertrophy in a 39 year old male patient prior to laser therapy.

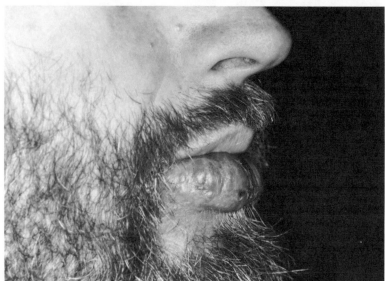

Fig. 5b. Reduction in size of the lower lip after two Nd:YAG laser treatments.

REFERENCES

1. Apfelberg,D.B., Maser,M.R., Lash,H., Rivers,J.: The Argon laser for cutaneous lesions. J.Am.Med.Assoc. 245, 2073-2075 (1981)
2. Landthaler,M., Haina,D., Waidelich,W., Braun-Falco,O.: Lasertherapy of venous lake (Bean-Walsh) and teleangiectases. J.Plast.Reconstr.Surg. (in press)
3. Reid,R., Muller,S.: Tattoo removal by CO_2 laser dermabrasion. Plast.Reconstr.Surg. 65, 717-728 (1980)
4. Baggish,M.S.: Carbon dioxide laser treatment for condylomata acuminata venereal infections. Obstet.Gynecol. 55, 711-715 (1980)
5. Lejeune,F.J., van Hoof,G., Gerard,A.: Impairment of skin graft take after CO_2 laser surgery in melanoma patients. Br.J.Surg. 67, 318-320 (1980)
6. Staehler,G.: Die externe Applikation von Neodym-YAG-Laserstrahlen in der Urologie. Urologe A. (Suppl.) 20, 323-327 (1981)
7. Hofstetter,A., Frank,F.: Der Neodym-YAG-Laser in der Urologie. Basel:Editiones Roche 1979
8. Goldmann,L., Nath,G., Schindler,G., Fidler,J., Rockwell,R.J.: High-power neodymium-YAG-laser surgery. Acta Dermatovenerol. (Stockholm) 53, 45-49 (1973)
9. Bahmer,F.A., Alzin,H.H.: Erste Erfahrungen mit dem Neodym-YAG-Laser in der Dermatologie. Akt. Dermatol. 9, 8-10 (1983)
10. Kozlov,A.P., Moskalik,K.G.: Pulsed laser radiation therapy of skin tumors. Cancer 46, 2172-2178 (1980)
11. Rothenberger,K., Pensel,J., Hofstetter,A., Keiditsch,E., Stern,J.: Dosierung der Neodym-YAG-Laserstrahlung zur endovesikalen Anwendung bei Blasentumoren. Urologe A (Suppl.) 20, 310-314 (1981)
12. Apfelberg,D.B., Kosek,J., Maser,M.R., Lash,H.: Histology of port wine stains following argon laser treatment. Br.J.Plast. Surg. 32, 232-237 (1979)
13. Keiditsch,E.: Histologische Grundlagen der endovesicalen Neodym-YAG-Laserbestrahlung. Urologe A (Suppl.) 20, 300-304 (1981)

CHAPTER 21

YAG LASER DERMABRASION OF TATTOOS

Principal Author:

Leon Goldman, M.D.
The Laser Treatment Center
The Laser Research Laboratory
The Jewish Hospital
Cincinnati, Ohio

YAG LASER DERMABRASION OF TATTOOS

Leon Goldman, M.D. and Wayne E. Bauman, M.D.
The Laser Treatment Center and The Laser Research Laboratory, The Jewish
Hospital, Cincinnati, Ohio.

ABSTRACT

For over 20 years, laser dermabrasion has been done for tattoos. The
value of laser dermabrasion has more selective specific effect on the
tattoo masses with lasers with the visible light range, such as the ruby,
argon and YAG. Other factors include narrow operating beams avoiding normal
tissues and short pulses also limiting the effect of the thermal coagulation
necrosis to the pigment area.

The current series of 32 tattoo patients treated with YAG lasers will
be reviewed.

For more than 20 years, lasers have been used in the dermabrasion of
tattoos.

1. Ruby 694.3 nm - pulsed

    A. 1962, normal mode Laser Laboratory Medical Center, University of
       Cincinnati

    B. 1965, Q switched mode Laser Laboratory Medical Center, University of
       Cincinnati (1,2)

    C. 1967, Q switched mode McLeod, Ritchie, Reid, Ferguson-Pell, Evans,
       Glasgow, Scotland (3)

2. Nd:YAG Laser 1060.0 nm CW

    A. 1969, Laser Laboratory Medical Center University of Cincinnati

    B. 1981, Laser Treatment Center, Jewish Hospital, Cincinnati

3. Argon Laser 488.0-514.5 nm CW

    A. 1973, Laser Laboratory Medical Center, University of Cincinnati

    B. 1976, Apfelberg, Maser, Lash, Palo Alto

    C. 1977, Ginsbach (5) Aachen, Germany

4. CO_2 laser 10,600 nm W

    A. 1978, Reid, Muller (6), Detroit

    B. 1980, Bailin (7), Ratz (8), Cleveland

The ruby laser, 694.3 nm then was used originally because there was
selected absorption in several colors of the tattoo. For the first time,
then dermabrasion with laser has a greater effect on those areas than on the
normal skin. The laser offered more than the other physical modalities used
for the treatment of tattoos, such as mechanical abrasion and chemical cauterization. The laser showed thermo-coagulation necrosis limited to color mass.
Small beams also limited the reaction to the selected treatment areas. Short
duration of the laser treatment also limited the reaction so that there was

Neodymium-YAG Laser in Medicine and Surgery, Joffe, Muckerheide, and Goldman, editors

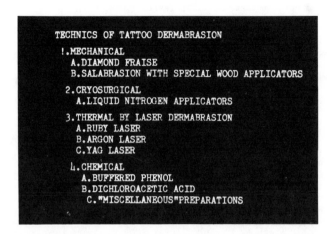

TECHNICS OF TATTOO DERMABRASION

!.MECHANICAL
  A.DIAMOND FRAISE
  B.SALABRASION WITH SPECIAL WOOD APPLICATORS

2.CRYOSURGICAL
  A.LIQUID NITROGEN APPLICATORS

3.THERMAL BY LASER DERMABRASION
  A.RUBY LASER
  B.ARGON LASER
  C.YAG LASER

4.CHEMICAL
  A.BUFFERED PHENOL
  B.DICHLOROACETIC ACID
  C."MISCELLANEOUS"PREPARATIONS

Figure 2. Technics of tattoo dermabrasion

little heat transmission or radiation to adjacent non-involved areas. The
ruby laser gave broad areas of reaction at 70 J/cm^2 2 nm/sec., 2.1 cm^2.
When Q switched ruby lasers were used, the duration was different from the
normal mode ruby laser which was 2 milliseconds. With the Q switched lasers,
the duration of the impact was in nanoseconds. Our initial experiments were
done with 20 nanoseconds. This made for immediate whitening, sharp localization of the laser impact to the target area. The difficulties were that the
target areas with our Q switched lasers, 1-1.5 mm, scarcely practical for
large tattoos. This difficulty with the apparatus and loss of funds meant
the cessation of these investigative studies. These studies with Q switched
ruby treatment of tattoos are being done in Glasgow, Scotland, now as
indicated. Our results with the laser dermabrasion of tattoos and those of
the investigators from Scotland were exhibited at the Third Annual Meeting of
The American Society of Laser Medicine and Surgery in January 1983.

Our experiments with the argon laser showed results which were not as
effective in spite of the selective absorption in the red and black. With
the argon laser, microsurgery was used with limitation of the reaction to
the tiny residual pigment masses.

As indicated, CO_2 laser dermabrasion was introduced by gynecologists,
Reid and Muller (6), and expanded in detail by Bailin, Ratz (8) and McBurney
(9). With the CO_2 laser, and absorption in all tissues, the value of the
laser was the small selective beam so that with moderate magnification or
through the CO_2 laser microscope, the impact could be localized to the tattoo
area and not affect the adjacent skin. This in unlike the reactions from the
mechanical abrasion with the high speed electrical diamond fraise and sala-
brasion or with chemical cauterization. Here, even normal tissues are
affected.

Recently, we had worked with the YAG (yttrium aluminum garnet) laser
1060 nm. This is in the near infrared. Years ago, we used the neodymium
YAG laser and the results were of interest with transmission through the
special fiber of Nath. We could get 90% transmission of the beam, making the
high output YAG laser a flexible instrument. The five patients treated 12
years ago, have been lost to observation. One was reported, recently, by
his family doctor to show minimal scarring of an extensive tattoo of the ankle.

With the current instrument, (Molectron), and with the fine gastric fiber (Fig. 2) which is used in endoscopy of the stomach and colon and for esophageal and pulmonary cancer, we are able to get localized thermocoagulation necrosis with deeper transmission so that deeper particles can be selectively removed. Our current series included 26 patients. This has been excellent on linear areas, dot areas, rather than on the broad color zones. Here too, the YAG laser has a selective effect on color, since impacts on normal skin have shown no reaction but immediate crusting developed when the beam moved to the tattoo. Outputs varied from 7-20 watts, pulses 6-10 seconds, pulse number 36 watts to 2394 J/cm^2.

With the technique suggested by Bailin and Ratz of curettement with peroxide and the continuous treatment advocated by Dixon, for deep penetration into the tissue, as with all forms of tattoo treatment, scarring does develop. Where extensive areas are treated at one time, the scarring may be hypertrophic and require long periods to flatten (Fig. 3 and 4). Post operative treatment has been various antibiotic creams; 2) sponging with wet dressings of diluted Burrows solution. Recently, with the technique of Dismukes, we have used 40-50% aqueous urea solution with daily pressure bandages with telfa. These pressure rolls are used to try to prevent the hypertrophic scarring from developing. The pressure rolls used consist of a folded bandage with adhesive over the treated area of the tattoo (Fig. 5 and 6).

The current series of patients include 32, two with extensive tattoos previously treated years ago and 30 as new patients. The observation period has varied from 6-24 months. Thirty-two patients have been treated over the past 2 years. Twenty-two have completed treatment with satisfactory results. In 16, three have hypertrophic scarring. At present, 3 have whitish ghosts with varying bits of retained pigment. Ten patients are still under therapy. Efforts are being made now to repair our Q switched YAG laser to use Q switched impacts which should be very effective.

COMMENT

As with our experience of laser dermabrasion of tattoos 20 years ago, the YAG laser also does offer help in the treatment of tattoos. The chief reaction has been hypertrophic scarring. Our incidence in this series of 32 patients with only 22 completed is 1% at present. Many of these scars may fade gradually in the future. This has been our experience in the past with our ruby laser treatment series. Our argon and CO_2 laser treatment series are too small to give any critical data, but some CO_2 laser treated patients have had heavy hypertrophic scarring. The YAG laser series however will continue and the value of our post operative programs will be available in several years.

The question of post laser scarring is now under investigation in our Laser Research Laboratory in connection with the burn scar program of the Shrine Burn Center at our University. Tissue culture studies of fibroblasts, injections of corticosteroids, antihistaminics, urea and pressure pads of plastic are being used. At present, for practical uses, injections of suspensions of corticosteroids and pressure pads are used in our patients with the laser treatment of port wine marks and of tattoos. The pressure pads are applied over topical medications. The pads are pieces of clear plastic so that the skin can be observed. These are shaped for the scars. The plastic bits are applied daily and secured with Blenederm 3M adhesive. They are used 24 hours a day for weeks and months. The thick scar after a period becomes soft and spongy and flattens. The current topical medication of 20-40% urea was suggested by the studies of Dismukes in his prevention of scarring in his long experience of the laser treatment of skin lesions. The mechanisms of urea suppression are not known. That is why urea is included in our tissue culture studies. The Q switched studies with the YAG laser are to be started shortly (Fig. 6).

REFERENCES:

1. Goldman L, Wilson R.G., Hornby P. and Meyers.R.G.: Radiation from a Q switched ruby laser: Effect of repeated impacts of power output of 10 megawatts on a tattoo on man. J. Invest. Derm. 44:69-70, 1965.

2. Yules F.B., Laub D.R., Honey R., Vassiliadis A. and Crowley L.: The effect of Q switched ruby laser radiation on dermal pigment in man. Arch. Surg. 95:179-182.

3. McLeod P.S., Ritchie A., Reid W.H., Ferguson-Pell and Evans J.H.: Q switched ruby laser treatment of black tattoos. Exhibit American Society Laser Medicine and Surgery, New Orleans, Jan. 1983.

4. Apfelberg D.B., Maser M.R., and Lash H.: Argon laser treatment of decorated tattoos. Brit. J. Plast. Surg.

5. Ginsbach, Gertrude. Personal communication.

6. Reid R. and Muller S. Tattoo removal by CO_2 laser dermabrasion. Plast. and Recon. Surg. 65:717-728, 1980.

7. Bailin P. Personal communication.

8. Ratz J. Personal communication.

9. McBurney E. Personnel communication.

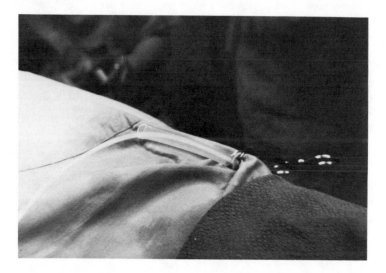

Figure 2. Holder at O.R. table for gastric fiber of YAG used in the YAG
laser dermabrasion of tattoos.

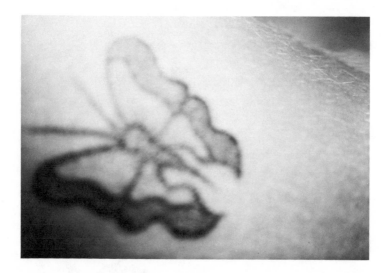

Figure 3. YAG laser dermabrasion of tattoo on forearm

A. butterfly tattooed on top of tattoo initials A I K in a 28
year old woman.

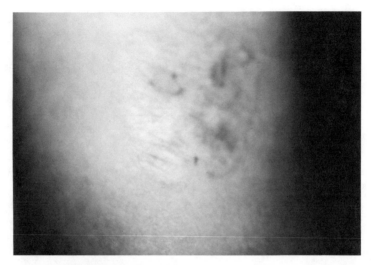

B. immediately after YAG laser gastric fiber dermabrasion
under local anesthesia.

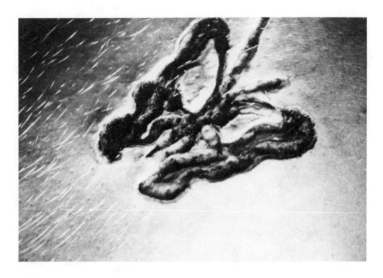

C. 4 months after YAG laser dermabrasion

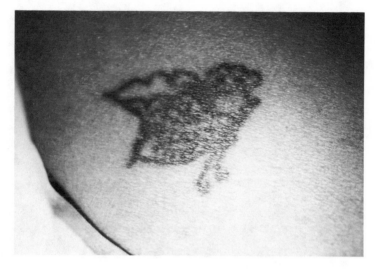

Figure 4. YAG laser dermabrasion of tattoo on shoulder of young woman

A. tattoo on shoulder before YAG laser dermabrasion

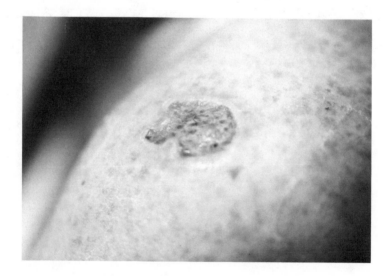

B. 3 weeks after treatment

193

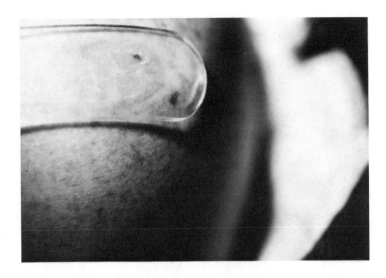

C. 4 months after treatment - showing melanosis under the
diascope

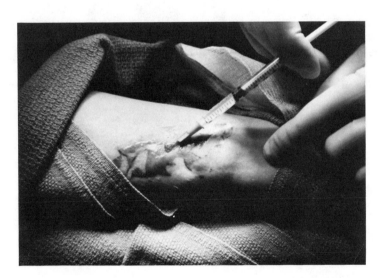

Figure 5. Injection of suspension of corticosteroids for hypertrophic
scarring following YAG laser dermabrasion of tattoo on forearm.

194

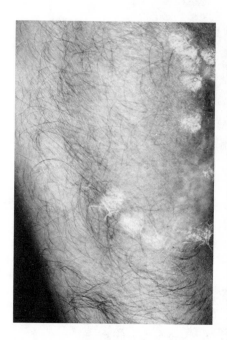

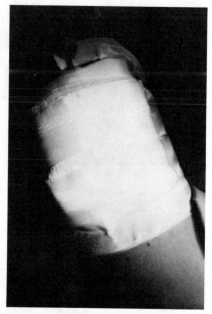

Figure 6. Q swtiched ruby laser
impacts for residual pigment spots
after ruby laser dermabrasion of
tattoo mark of forearm, 1969.

Figure 7. Pressure bandages after
laser dermabrasion of tattoos to
attempt to prevent and to treat
hypertrophic scarring.

CHAPTER 22

EVALUATION OF COOLING TECHNIQUES FOR THE PROTECTION OF THE

EPIDERMIS DURING Nd:YAG LASER IRRADIATION OF THE SKIN

Principal Author:
A.J. Welch, Ph.D.
Biomedical Engineering Program
University of Texas at Austin
Austin, Texas

EVALUATION OF COOLING TECHNIQUES FOR THE
PROTECTION OF THE EPIDERMIS DURING ND-YAG
LASER IRRADIATION OF THE SKIN

A.J. Welch, PhD., M. Motamedi, MS., A. Gonzalez, MS.MD.,
Biomedical Engineering Program, University of Texas at
Austin, Texas 78712

INTRODUCTION

Argon ion lasers have been used for approximately 15 years in the
treatment of several cutaneous lesions. The lesions involving blood vessel
abnormalities such as Port Wine Stain, capillary cavernous haemangiomas and
telangiectasias form the group most frequently treated by Argon Laser. Less
common is the use of lasers in the removal of tattoos and occasionally in inflamatory nevoid or fibrogranuloamtous processes (1). Port Wine Stain (PWS)
is the most frequent dermatological entity treated with Argon Laser and its
usefulness has been well recognized (2-4).

A PWS treatment is considered successful if blanching of the lesion
is achieved without leaving scars or atrophy. The ultimate laser effect in
whitening of the lesion has been described by Solomon et al. (5) as "a nonspe-
cific coagulation necrosis effect in the collagen and elastic fibers of the
upper dermis followed by the formation of a cicatrix." This fibrosis diminishes
the number and the diameter of the ectatic vessels resulting in reduction of the
amount of blood in the dermis thus turning the skin surface lighter. The
healing of the photocoagulated area is rapid and is helped by the skin appendages (hair follicles and sweat glands) that seem to be impervious to Argon
Laser irradiation (1,6). Success in the Argon treatment of PWS has been reported
in 59 to 75 percent of the cases (2,4,7). Failure, however, is still seen in
many patients, due to scarring of the irradiated area which occurs in nine to
thirteen percent of the treatments. In recent years, various lasers have been
used in the treatment of tattoos. Ideally the laser light is differentially
absorbed in the tattoo pigment which removes the pigment deposited in the dermis
and leaves little or no scar (8,9).

Scarring of the irradiated skin is only a continuation of the healing
process, but with an exaggerated formation of fibrous tissue that virtually
replaces the normal dermal structures. There are several reasons for this un-
desired outcome: the absorption of the Argon light in the first millimeter of
tissue produces "extensive thermal necrosis of the entire epidermis and the first
millimeter of dermis" (5,10). Since the basal layer of the epidermis and the
uppermost papillary layer of the dermis are the keys for skin restoration,
anamolous hypertrophic scarring is not unusual in these cases. The number of
ectatic vessels and their fullness (i.e., volume of blood) is also a factor for
hypertrophic scarring as described by Noe et al. (2). Pink lesions with minimal
percent fullness have less blood to absorb the Argon light than dark high blood
volume lesions. They suggest that for pink lesions more energy is absorbed by
the surrounding tissue which causes more damage to cells, collagen and elastic
fibers than in the darker lesions.

Gilchrest et al. (11) lowered by 57 percent the incidence of scarring
by chilling the skin with a bag of ice prior to irradiation. They hoped to
produce a dark tone in the PWS before irradiation, by increasing the amount of

Neodymium-YAG Laser in Medicine and Surgery, Joffe, Muckerheide, and Goldman, editors

stagnated blood in the ectatic vessels. This, however, was not the case. Biopsies showed a reduction in the volume of blood in the skin. Nevertheless, the cooling did reduce scarring. They concluded that "reducing the tissue temperature may significantly widen the safety margin in laser treated skin and so avoid scarring."

Surface cooling techniques should improve the outcome of laser treatment of PWS and tattoo removal. Our research has had two main objectives. First, to evaluate the usefullness of three different cooling methods as follows: precooling of the skin surface with ice and water before laser irradiation, cooling with chilled water while irradiating the skin and, cooling with freon gas during irradiation. Second, to compare the effectiveness of Argon and ND-YAG lasers to produce photocoagulation of the dermis while protecting the epidermis with a surface cooling technique.

THEORY

Thermal insult of skin is the result of an evaluation of tissue temperature above a threshold value for a finite period of time. Both the temperature and duration of irradiation are important in determining the degree of thermal insult. When laser light is absorbed in the tissue, the light energy is converted to heat which creates a temperature rise in the tissue. Temperature dependent rate reactions lead to protein denaturation and coagulation. This process can be described in terms of 1) a heat source term due to absorption of laser irradiation, 2) a three dimensional temperature field and, 3) a rate process of damage (see Figure 1). The temperature field is computed using the heat conduction equation (12) and damage is estimated by a rate process model developed by Henriques (13). Although the rate process is an involved process, we assume there exists a critical coagulation temperature, T_c, such that coagulation occurs at all points in the tissue that have a temperature equal to or greater than T_c.

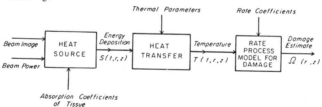

Figure 1: A mathematical representation of thermal damage of tissue is depicted as a) light conversion to heat (heat source), b) creation of temperature field (heat transfer), c) temperature dependent rate reaction (rate process model for damage).

In this research our primary concern is the effect of surface cooling procedure on the laser induced temperature field and the conditions to reach T_c. Because of the low absorption properties of skin for ND-YAG irradiation, the heat source is distributed throughout epidermis and dermis. Figure 2 shows the general influence of each cooling modality on temperature and tissue damage for a fixed irradiation condition. Values are relative to a "non-cooled" tissue response. In case A, the combination of the heat source in the epidermis and lack of heat transfer at the surface cause suprathreshold damage in the epidermis.

In case B, precooling lowers both the temperature of the dermis and epidermis. Thus laser power must be increased to compensate for the drop in tissue temperature due to precooling. In case C, there is no initial change in dermal temperature but the epidermis temperature is lowered due to the chilled water temperature. Heat from the epidermis source term is efficiently removed by conduction of heat from skin to water and forced convection of the flow of chilled water. The rapid cooling required a higher irradiation power than in case A to achieve the coagulation threshold, T_c, in the dermis.

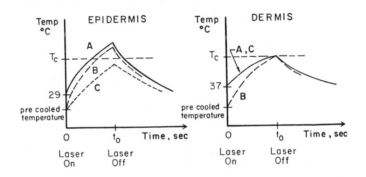

Figure 2: An illustration of temperature profiles in the epidermis and dermis during and after laser irradiation. Case A is normal, uncooled tissue, Case B is precooled tissue, and Case C is chilled water cooled tissue. In each case the power of the laser is adjusted to produce threshold coagulation in the dermis.

MATERIAL AND METHODS

The lasers used in these experiments were an Argon Ion Laser (Coherent Model CR-5) capable of a maximum power output of 2.5 watts in the all-lines modality, and a CW ND-YAG Laser (Holobeam Laser Inc. Model 2660-IR) with a maximum output of up to 100 watts.

A fiber optic and collimating lens system was used to deliver the laser beam onto the animal's skin. The half divergence angle at the output of the optical system was 3.25 degrees for ND-YAG and 2.3 degrees for Argon. The energy loss through the fiber optic system was 15 percent for ND-YAG and 20 percent for the Argon laser. the e^{-2} spot diameter was 2.2 mm (area-3.8 mm^2) for the ND-YAG and 1.6 mm (area-2.0 mm^2) for the Argon laser.

White mini pigs weighing 8-10 kilograms were used in the experiment. The animals were anesthesized with chlorpromazine (Thorazine) and pentobarbitol sodium (Nembutal). The flanks were shaved, a grid was drawn on the flanks and the tissue within each grid was irradiated as follows: First, for ND-YAG laser irradiation - Method 1: No cooling treatment (for control), eight to fifteen burns were made for several power settings varying from 10-30 watts and time exposure from 0.5 to 2 seconds to produce small but visible burns. Method 2: Precool with ice - a plastic bag with ice and water at 0°C was placed on the skin for 5 minutes, lowering the skin surface temperature to 20°C. The irradiation was carried out using output powers and exposure times which produced visible burns. Method 3: Freon Gas - compressed commercial freon spray (Circuit Cooler, G.C. Electronics) was used during the irradiation. The nozzle of the freon can was kept at 8 to 16 centimeters away from the skin depending on laser irradiation time. It was held closer for the short exposures and further for the longer exposure times. Method 4: Chilled water - cooled water (0.4 to 1.0 degrees Centigrade) was spread directly on the area being irradiated for the duration of the irradiation. Power and exposure time were selected to produce small but visible burns. The same cooling modalities were used during Argon laser irradiation tests. The incident Argon power ranged from 0.5 to 2.0 watts for exposure times of 2 to 25 seconds. A list of experimental irradiations is presented in Tables I and II (see page 5).

In addition, one pig was tattooed with a dark blue pigment. The ink was injected into the dermal layer according to usual tattoo procedure. Normal and tattooed tissue was irradiated with both the ND-YAG and Argon lasers. There were fifteen lesions formed with the ND-YAG laser using 2 to 10 watts for 0.5 to 2 seconds. Eighteen lesions were formed with the Argon laser using 1 to 2 watts for 2 to 40 seconds. During each irradiation one of the cooling procedures was tested.

The animals were sacrificed an hour after the last irradiation. The irradiated skin was removed and held straight during the histologic preparation. Fixation was carried out with Bouin's Fluid, after which every burn was split in two halves with the cross section plane passing vertically through the center of the burn. Dioxane was used for dehydration and the parafin embedded tissues were sectioned at 6 micrometers and stained with H & E.

RESULTS

One hundred twenty burns out of the one hundred eighty-four burns were suitable for measurement and classification. Generally all the burns were micro-scopically similar. The thermal insult produced a coagulative necrosis, mani-fested by Pyknosis, Karyorrhexis and cell nucleus vacuolization. The epidermal cells showed the worse damage which extended deep into the dermis. Necrotic vessels appeared with clotted or crenated erythrocytes along with distorted endothelium. The collagen and elastic fibers appeared swollen and more eosi-nophilic. Very little edema was present and no inflamatory signs (i.e., leucocytic migration) were seen. No blisters developed in any of the burns. The skin appendages - hair follicles and sweat glands - showed generally the same necrotic changes, they did not seem to be more susceptible nor more impervious to the laser light. Typical damage results for the cooling pro-cedure and various exposure conditions are listed in Tables I and II (see Page 5).

Evaluation of each cooling procedure was based on a criteria of coagulation of blood vessels in the dermis and minimal damage to the epidermis. The precooling technique using ice water did not show any improvement over the control. Higher power and longer exposure durations were required for the desired level of dermal damage. However, these levels caused excessive epidermal damage. In the other two cooling modalities, freon and chilled water applied during irradiation, some positive results were seen. Tables I and II summarize the epidermal protection results.

TABLE I

Typical Exposure Conditions and Histological Results
for ND-YAG Irradiation of Normal Pig Skin

Cooling Modality	Power (watts)	Exposure Time (seconds)	Energy Density (joules/cm^2)	Percent of Damage		
				Epidermis	Dermis	Fat
Control	25	2	1315	100	100	50
Control	30	2	1578	100	100	100
Pre-cooling	25	2	1315	100	34	0
Pre-cooling	30	2	1578	100	100	0
Freon	20	2	1052	0	72	0
Freon	30	2	1578	0	80	0
Chilled water	30	2	1578	0	62	0
Chilled water	35	3	2762	0	67	0

TABLE II

Typical Exposure Conditions and Histological Results for Argon
Irradiation of Normal Pig Skin

Cooling Modality	Power (watts)	Exposure Time (seconds)	Energy Density (joules/cm^2)	Percent of Damage		
				Epidermis	Dermis	Fat
Control	1	7	348	100	45	0
Precooling	1	10	497	100	13	0
Freon	1	12	597	100	22	0
Chilled water	1.8	22	1969	100	47	0

The protective action of these fluids was manifested by a normal, nondamaged epidermis (and in a few cases undamaged upper dermis), leaving the burn confined to the lower dermis and sometimes touching the subcutaneous fat.

In the group of burns made with ND-YAG laser, 28 percent of the burns cooled by freon displayed an undamaged epidermis. The same protection was seen in 100 percent of the burns cooled with chilled water. Due to technical problems, the number of burns produced by Argon laser was greatly diminished and only in one out of four freon-cooled burns (25 percent) was the protective effect to the epidermis seen. (see Table III).

TABLE III

Selected Burns of Normal Pig Skin

Modality	# of Burns (ND-YAG)	No Damage to Epidermis	# of Burns (Argon)	No Damage to Epidermis
Control	18	0	18	0
Precooling	12	0	5	0
Freon	14	4	4	1
Chilled Water	8	8	2	0

Tables IV and V show the epidermal protection results for the tattoed pig.

TABLE IV

Typical Exposure Conditions and Histological Results of
ND-YAG Irradiated Tattoos

Cooling Modality	Power (watts)	Exposure Time (seconds)	Energy Density (Joules/cm^2)	Percent of Damage		
				Epidermis	Dermis	Fat
Control	3	1	79	100	67	0
Precooling	2	2	105	100	64	0
Freon	3	1	79	0	76	0
Chilled Water	2	2	105	0	52	0

TABLE V

Typical Exposure Conditions and Histological Results of
Argon Irradiated Tattoos

Cooling Modality	Power (watts)	Exposure Time (seconds)	Energy Density (Joules/cm^2)	Percent of Damage		
				Epidermis	Dermis	Fat
Control	1.0	7.0	348	100	76	0
Precooling	1.8	5.5	492	100	39	0
Freon	1.8	3.0	268	100	25	0
Chilled Water	1.8	25.0	2237	100	64	0

DISCUSSION

Argon Ion Laser treatment of Port Wine Stains can leave a permanent
scar in up to 13 percent of the cases (1) and skin atrophy in 6 percent of them
(4). Both phenomena are the result of a coagulative necrosis of the tissue
followed by a formation of a cicatrix (10). The injury to the epidermis is
crucial in the development of the fibrotic scar (14). It seems, then, reasonable
to protect the epidermis from the thermal insult in order to decrease the
incidence of scarring. Gilchrest, et al. (11) significantly reduced the
incidence of scars by cooling the skin with ice before irradiation. They believed
lowering the skin surface temperature would avoid scarring.

In this experiment involving normal pig skin, the ice cooling before
irradiation did not show improvement over the control with respect to damage to
the epidermis. Theoretically this cooling procedure lowers the temperature of
both the epidermis and the dermis. Thus to reach a critical temperature in the
lower dermis for damage required proportionally higher levels of irradiation.
It is possible that a shorter time of application (enough to only cool down the
epidermis but not the dermis) may give positive results.

The freon method developed in this lab showed good results in 28.5
percent of the cases. There was no involvement of the epidermis while producing deep dermal burns. The technique, however, needs some improvements
because in some cases the skin surface was momentarily frozen and in others the
freon jet was not sufficient to properly cool the skin surface. A more
controlled means of freon application should provide effective cooling of the
epidermis.

The best results were obtained with the chilled water modality (100
percent positive results). These results are probably due to a more constant and
uniform rate of cooling of the surface. The water temperature was held between
0.4 and 1.0°C and the flow rate was basically the same in all cases. Under
these conditions, heat was conducted from skin to water at a rate fast enough to
keep the surface temperature under the damage threshold level. While the

epidermis was protected, the dermis was damaged due to dissipation of heat which resulted in temperatures beyond the threshold level.

In the tattooed pig, due to higher absorption of light by pigmented tissue, a significantly smaller energy density was needed to produce the same depth of damage as in normal tissue. The results show that cooling the skin during laser irradiation protects epidermis and reduces the extent of damage to the pigmented tissue the same way as for normal tissue. The reduction in power for the ND-YAG laser is approximately 70 percent. This reduction is due not only to the high absorption properties of the pigment in the tattoo ink, but also a reduction in reflection of light at the surface of the tissue. In turn the apparent reduction in reflected energy may be due to a reduction of back scattering of the laser light in the tissue.

Comparing the performance of the two lasers in this experiment, it seems that ND-YAG lasers could be used in the treatment of PWS and tattoos. Application of ND-YAG in treatment of PWS may have two advantages. First, ND-YAG laser penetrates about 2½ times deeper than Argon. This may help in the treatment of those PWS in which the majority of the vessels are in the base of the dermis. According to Ohmari and Huang, 50 percent of the PWS's fit this category and the Argon laser is of no use due to its shallow penetration (6,10). Second, when used with a suitable cooling procedure, ND-YAG laser can produce dermal burns, while leaving the epidermis unharmed. One must caution, however, that these advantages were seen when experimenting with normal skin.

CONCLUSIONS

1. Protection of the epidermis during laser irradiation of skin can be achieved effectively with the chilled water cooling method described here.

2. The freon gas modality could be of similar effectiveness if the application technique is improved.

3. Under the conditions described in this work the precooling technique using ice and water for five minutes prior to the irradiation did not improve the epidermis protection.

4. The ND-YAG laser can be used to photocoagulate tissue deep in the dermis, where the Argon laser cannot reach.

5. Chilled water and freon gas techniques for cooling of the skin surface worked better when coupled with the ND-YAG than with the Argon laser.

6. The cooling techniques described in this paper in conjunction with ND-YAG irradiation of cutaneous tissue may prove useful in the treatment of PWS and removal of tattoos.

REFERENCES

1. Apfelberg, et al., "The Argon Laser for Cutaneous Lesions." JAMA, 245(20):2073-2075 (1981).

2. Noe, J.M. et al., "Port Wine Stains and the Response to Argon Laser Therapy: Successful Treatment and the Predictive Role of Color, Age, and Biopsy." Plastic and Reconstructive Surgery, 65(2):130-136 (1980).

3. Apfleberg, D.B., et al., "Histology of Port Wine Stains Following Argon Laser Treatment." Br. Jl. of Plastic Surgery, 32:232-237 (1979).

4. Goldman, L., Dreffer, R., "Laser Treatment of Extensive Mixed Cavernous and Port Wine Stains." Arch. Dermatolo., 113:504-505 (1979).

5. Solomon, H., et al., "Histopathology of the Laser Treatment of Port Wine Lesions." Jl. Invest. Dermatol., 50(2):141-146 (1968).

6. Apfelberg, D.B., Maser, M.F., Lash, H., "Argon Laser Treatment of Cutaneous Vascular Abnormalities: Progress Report." Annals of Plastic Surgery, 1(1):14-18 (1978).

7. Gilchrest, B.A., Rosen, S., and Noe, J.M., "Chilling Port Wine Stains Improves the Response to Argon Laser Therapy." Plastic and Reconstructive Surgery, 69(2):278-283 (1982).

8. Apfelbery, D.B.m et al., "Pathophysiology and Treatment of Decorative Tattoos with Reference to Argon Laser Treatment" Clinics in Plastic Surgery, 7(3):369-377 (1980).

9. Arellano, C.R., et al., "Tattoo Removal: Comparative Study of six Methods in the Pig" Plastic and Reconstructive Surgery, 70(6):699-703.

10. Ohmori, S., and Huang, C., "Recent Progress in the Treatment of Port Wine Stains by Argon Laser: Some Observations of the Prognostic Value of Relative Spectro-Reflectance (RSR) and the Histological Classification of the Lesions." Br. Jl. of Plastic Surgery, 34:249-257 (1981).

11. Gilchrest, B.A.. et al., "Chilling Port Wine Stains Improves the Response to Argon Laser Therapy" Plastic and Reconstructive Surgery, 69(2):278-283 (1982).

12. Mainster, M.A., et al. "Transient Thermal Behavior in Biological Systems" Bulletin of Mathematical Biophysics, 32 303-314 (1970).

13. Henriques, F.F., "Studies of Thermal Injury: V. Predictability of Thermally Induced Rate Process Leading to Epidermal Injury," Archives of Pathology, 43:489-502 (1947).

14. Anderson, R.R., and Parrish, J.A., "Microvasculatore Can Be Selectively Damaged Using Dye Lasers: A Basic Theory and Experimental Evidence in Human Skin." Lasers in Surgery and Medicine, 1:263-276 (1981).

ACKNOWLEDGMENT: This work was sponsored in part by a grant from Promed Inc.

CHAPTER 23

INSTRUMENTATION AND SAFETY ASPECTS FOR THE SURGICAL

APPLICATION OF THE Nd:YAG LASER

Principal Author:

F. Frank
MBB-Angewandte Technologie GmbH
P.O.B. 801168
8000 München W., Germany

Instrumentation and Safety Aspects for the Surgical Application of the
Nd:YAG Laser

Frank, F.
MBB-Angewandte Technologie GmbH P.O.B. 801168, 8000 München W. Germany

in collaboration with

Bailer,P.[1], Beck,O.[2], Böwering,R.[3], Hofstetter,A.[3]
1) Frauenklinik vom Roten Kreuz München
2) Neurochirurg. Klinik, Klinikum Großhadern der Universität München
3) Urolog. Abteilung, Städt. Krankenhaus Thalkirchnerstraße München

ABSTRACT

The Nd:YAG laser has become a coagulation instrument, which has found
acceptance in interdisciplinary surgery. The main contributors are its highly
efficient coagulation capability in interaction with tissue and the fact that
the Nd:YAG laser beam can be transmitted by means of a simple quartz-glass
fiber. Appropriate systems and instruments for transmission and operation have
been developed for the various applications in neurosurgery, pulmonology, gastroenterology, urology, gynaecology and dermatology. Operation methods in open and
endoscopic surgery under use of several hand held devices and flexible as well
as rigid endoscopes are being demonstrated by clinical examples of application.
Necessary safety regulations are being explained.

INTRODUCTION

Due to the low absorption and high scattering effects in tissue, the radiation of the Nd:YAG laser, which lies in the near infrared range of λ = 1.06 µ,
leads to a deep and homogeneous coagulation effect. Combined with the possibility to transmit the Nd:YAG laser beam by means of quartz-glass fibers, the
Nd:YAG laser has become a coagulation instrument of interdisciplinary application possibilities. The contactless treatment and the fact that blood and
lymphatic vessels are coagulated at least for a certain period, led to successful applications especially with regard to tumor surgery.

LASER SYSTEM

For routine clinical use the mediLas Nd:YAG laser made by Messerschmitt-
Bölkow-Blohm, Angewandte Technologie GmbH, has proven very successful.
The system consists of a mobile desk housing with an operating console. The
desk accommodates the electric circuitry,the control unit, and the cooling
system. The laser head is attached to the console by an articulating arm and
houses all the optical components of the Nd:YAG laser, i.e. the crystal, pump
lamps, resonator mirrors, and lamp casing. It also has a pilot laser beam
emitting low-power radiation in the visible range. The pilot light is positioned concentrically with respect to the therapeutic beam. Both are transmitted
to the target area through a flexible fiber-optic light guide. The pilot light
thus marks the target point for the therapeutic beam. The light guide is
fitted to the laser head by means of a plug in which the optical coupling
system is integrated. The operating console permits digital selection of the
pulse intensity and duration. Integrated power measurement and indicator units
are included. A printer documents the indicated data for each laser pulse.
The mains unit contains all the electrical supply elements. The current for the
pump lamps and thus the laser power is regulated under thyristor control.
Further electronic switching and monitoring elements allow largely automatic

running of the system. The lamp casing, the lamps, and the crystal are cooled with water. The dual-circuit cooling system, comprising flow monitors and magnetic valves, is housed in the cooling unit. The system fulfils all the requirements for clinical application: ease of operation, small size, and a high degree of mobility. The safety devices conform to both German and international laser-safety specifications (VBG 93, IEC Draft, FDA Health and Safety Act).

ENDOSCOPIC APPLICATION

Of the various indications for the use of Nd:YAG laser in medicine, applications in the endoscopic field have reached an essential importance. Applications must be differentiated according to utilization of flexible and rigid endoscopes.

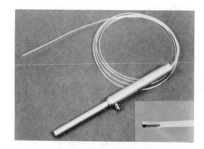

Fig. 1. Nd.YAG laser light guide with coaxial gas cooling

Using flexible endoscopes, transmission of the laser beam is effected by means of a light guide with coaxial gas cooling. The gas enters at the light guide connector where the optic coupling system is integrated. At the distal end an appropriate nozzle is adapted to provide for an efficient rinsing and cooling of the tip of the light guide. (See Fig. 1.)

In gastroenterology all routine diagnostic instruments are applied without any modification. The light guide is passed directly through the working channel and can be moved in the distal direction. The application of Nd:YAG laser in gastroenterology is suitable for staunching of bleedings from esophageal varices as well as for treatment of ulcers and Mallory-Weiss tears. Tumor treatments in the upper and lower gastrointestinal tract are additional indications. For the intervention only conscious sedation is necessary.[1,2] Owing to the effective staunching of bleedings immediately after localization further surgical interventions can be undertaken under controlled conditions. Additionally, an efficient renunciation of blood-conserves is reached.

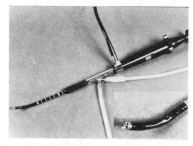

Fig. 2. Flexible Endoscope with Nd:YAG laser light guide

In pulmonology all routine diagnostic instruments can be applied. Flexible bronchoscopes are being used as well as rigid instruments with distal fiber movement.[3,4,5] The intervention is performed under outpatient conditions. The instruments are introduced nasally and orally after local anaesthesia. The Nd:YAG laser is applied to recanalize endobronchial and endotracheal stenoses as well as for the resection of bronchial tumors.

In a special flexible endoscopic system with a lumen of only 4,5 mm the light guide fiber is passed through the working channel simultaneously with fluid rinsing. 14 (See Fig. 2.)

This instrument has proven itself especially suitable for hypophysectomy as well as for the treatment of tumors of the hypophysis with Nd:YAG laser. It is introduced transsphenoidally and its localization can be controlled through the operating microscope or by means of an image intensifier. Owing to the coagulation effect in the hypophysis' tissue such interventions are significantly facilitated, since bleedings hardly ever occur.

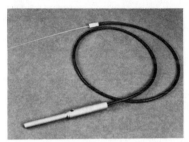

The various rigid endoscopes are used with liquid-rinsed light guides. The rinsing is connected directly to the endoscopic system. A special spring mechanism allows the fiber to be shifted in the distal direction. (See Fig. 3.)

For the treatment of tumors in the urogenital system several endoscopic laser instruments are available 6.

For outpatient treatment of small bladder tumors, stage TIS and T1, the instrument is composed of a conventional urethrocystoscope sheath of 19-21 French, a standard observation optic with variable viewing angles and a special laser

Fig. 3. Nd:YAG laser light guide with liquid rinsing

cystoscope insert. In this arrangement the light guide is passed directly through the ureter-catheter channel of the special Albarran instrument.7 (See Fig. 4.) The proximal end of the light guide can be bent to an angle of

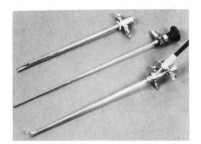
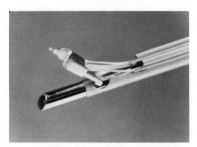

Fig. 4. Nd:YAG laser urethrocystoscope w. Albarran insert

Fig. 5. Albarran lever in detail

up to 80° with the aid of the Albarran lever, designed in a way that the fiber end is affixed in a protected manner. In addition, the fiber end can be distally moved in order to permit exact distance adjustment to the area irradiated. (See Fig. 5.)

For clinical interventions on larger tumors and for laser irradiation of the tumor bed after electroresection a 24 French resection sheath is used instead of the sheath just described. The greater rinsing effect achieved leads to an efficient irradiation even when bleedings occur. The mobility of the fiber end resulting from the incorporated capability to bend and to shift the light guide allows reaching and irradiation of tumors in an optimal manner located at any point on the bladder wall.

Bladder tumors up to the size of a cherry can be totally necrotized with the Nd:YAG laser. For larger tumors a combined treatment with laser and TUR is recommended.

Immediately after Nd:YAG laser irradiation a whitish discoloration is visual evidence of the deep and homogeneous coagulation effect. Since only negligible bleedings will occur, catheters are not necessary and, thus, nosocomial infections are being avoided.8,9,10 Within four days the necrotic tumor sloughs off. Some weeks later revascularization and scar formation follows.

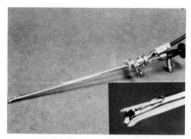

Fig. 6. Endoscope for Nd:YAG laser application within the urethra

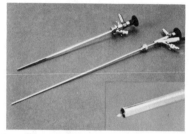

Fig. 7. Two-piece pyeloscope for Nd:YAG laser treatment within the ureter

For irradiation of tumors within the urethra, use can be made of a modified cystoscope sheath of 15.5 French with a lateral opening on its proximal end. The fiber is passed through the sheath together with the observation optic and can be moved in the distal direction.11 (See Fig. 6.)

For example, condylomatas in the urethra can be completely denaturated by Nd:YAG laser irradiation. When the tumor has sloughed off the base is irradiated as a prophylactic measure against recurrence.

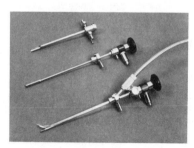

Fig. 8. Nd:YAG laser encephaloscope and viewing obturator

ted.14

A two-piece pyeloscope of 9-11 French has been designed for tumor treatment within the lower part of the ureter. Fiber and viewing optics are being inserted into the part of the instrument which will be moved into the ureter.12,13 (See Fig. 7.)

A special laser-encephaloscope to permit controlled movement of the distal end of the flexible fiber has been created for the endoscopic Nd:YAG laser intervention in the ventricle system and for perforation of brain cysts. (See Fig. 8.) After introduction of the sheath of 14 French under visual control the Albarran attachment with the fiber will be inser-

210

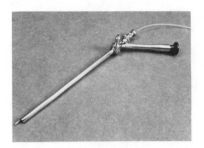

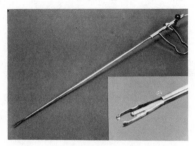

Fig. 9. Laparoscope with Nd:YAG
laser light guide

Fig. 10. Laparoscope insert for tubal
sterilization

For laparoscopic application of the Nd:YAG laser in gynaecology a laser
light guide with a co-axial gasflow can be adapted to the routine operation-
laparoscopes. (See Fig. 9.) Owing to the homogeneous coagulation effect the
Nd:YAG laser is also successfully applied to tuba sterilization. The distal
foreceps of this laparoscope insert ensure a permanent obturation of the
ovular tuba.15 (See Fig. 10.)

APPLICATION IN OPEN SURGERY

For all operations on an exposed area or for external applications, various
operation handpieces have been designed.

The focussing handpiece utilizes an interchangeable optic. Focus points of
minimal 0,4 mm diameter can be achieved. By altering the irradiation distance,
both, the power density and the diameter of the treatment area can be varied.
(See Fig. 11.)

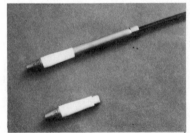

Fig. 11. Nd:YAG laser focussing handpiece w.interchangeable optic

In neurosurgery the focussing handpiece is used for the removal of meningiomas. Irradiation by Nd:YAG laser is
indicated, if complications are to be
expected due to locations or vasculari-
zation.16 For example the preparation of
a meningioma with sinus infiltration is
facilitated by the Nd:YAG laser irradiation causing the tumor to shrink. The
thorough coagulation of the tumor remains in the sinus wall acts as an
efficient prophylactic measure against
relapses and, in some cases, spares the
patient a risky sinusplasty. As a rule,
transfusions become unnecessary due to
little loss of blood during the operation.

The focussing handpiece is also used in urology for irradiation of tumors
at the outer genital tract. For example, condylomata of the fossa navicularis
can easily be coagulated by Nd:YAG laser irradiation. An inspection of the
urethra should follow.17,18

The possibility to alter the energy density by varying the irradiation
distance has proven advantageous especially in dermatologic indications. Any
spot size is possible ranging from large areas all the way to tiny spots.
Treatment with the aid of the Nd:YAG laser is indicated in a great number of
virological transformations as well as tumors of the skin, like basiliomas,
morbus Bowen and actinic keratoses.19 Removing warts with the Nd:YAG laser
avoids the resection of a large surrounding area, as it is indicated in case of
conventional treatment with the scalpel. After removal of the coagulated
tissue healing with a good cosmetic result is ensured.

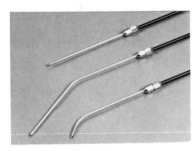 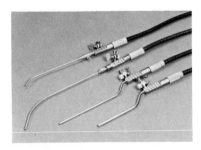

Fig. 12. Handapplicators with gas coo- Fig. 13. Handapplicators with liquid
     led Nd:YAG laser light guide   rinsed Nd:YAG laser light guide

For interventions under the operating microscope, simple handapplicators
of different shapes have been designed for unrestricted three-dimensional free-
hand manipulation. Systems with gas or liquid rinsing are available. (See Fig.
12,13.)

There is a vast number of neurosurgical indications for these instruments
particularly in those cases when the removal of a tumor can be expected to
cause complications due to its location. The slim configuration of the instruments ensures unimpaired vision. These microsurgical instruments have proven
helpful for treatment of sphenoid wing meningioma, cervico-cranial meningiomas,
tumors in the posterior fossa, and in the sella region.

All of the instruments presented have been created to complement the mediLas
YAG laser made by Messerschmitt-Bölkow-Blohm, Angewandte Technologie GmbH.
Many of these instruments are either patented or internationally registered
for patents.

SAFETY ASPECTS

The prerequisite for the use of high-powered lasers for clinical interventions in medicine is complete safety for the patient, the doctor and the auxiliary personnel in respect of laser radiation hazards. The aim of clinical laser
therapy is controlled denaturation of organic tissue. However, at the same time
it is essential to ensure that the radiation intensity outside the treatment
region is attenuated to the extent that there is no risk to the doctor in
charge or to his assistants. Moreover, there must be adequate protections
against any radiation unintentionally emitted outside the field of operation.

Improper use of laser equipment can result in thermal damage to the eye as
well as in skin damage. In case of lasers emitting in the visible and near

infrared region between 400 and 1400 nm like the Nd:YAG laser the main danger
is that of retina damage because of the transparency of the lens of the eye.

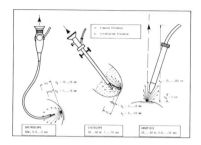 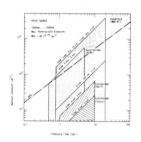

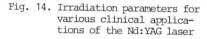

Fig. 14. Irradiation parameters for
various clinical applica-
tions of the Nd:YAG laser

Fig. 15. Radiation exposure at the eye
for surgical instruments and
operational conditions for
Nd:YAG laser applications

The use of the Nd:YAG laser in endoscopic and open surgery necessitates a
number of different safety precautions corresponding to the different techniques and irradiation parameters. (See Fig. 14.) For the safe use of laser
equipment the draft of the International Electrotechnical Commission (IEC),
"Radiation safety of laser products, equipment classification, requirements
and user's guide" can be considered obligatory. The IEC draft defines the maximum permissible exposure for the eye and the skin, for the whole spectrum of
laser instruments. The stimulated MPE values depend on whether the instrument
in question is a continuous-wave laser or a pulsed laser and on whether the
laser source is a point or an extended source; they also vary of course as a
function of wavelength and exposure time.

Different endoscopes and several handpieces had been experimentally tested
in order to measure the radiation exposure to the eye caused by backscattering.
The gained data had been compared with the MPE values. The irradiation parameters were varied in correspondence to the clinical procedure.20

When using the rigid laser cystoscopes, in the worst possible case, e.g.
with a viewing distance of 8 mm, an irradiation distance of 3 mm and a power
of 50 W, the radiation exposure is still clearly below the MPE value.

In case of the gastroscope and bronchoscope, especially with an exposure
time longer than 0·5 sec., radiation exposure values occur that are above the
permissible level. For this reason the eyepiece should always be fitted with
a filter such as KG 3 Schott filter 2 mm thick with a transmission coefficient
of 10^{-3} for the Nd:YAG laser wavelength.

For interventions with the surgical handpiece or the hand applicators, in
which the surgeon has a wide visual range from which to view, some 25 cm, the
radiation exposure limit for the eye is considerably exceeded even with a
initial laser output of 50 W. Although the exposure to backscattered radiation
at a distance of 1 m is certainly below the MPE value, radiation can escape
into the operating room, especially when the handpiece is used without due
care, and thus, all the people present at the operation must wear protective

glasses. Commercially available glasses with a transmission density of 7 are
also adequate at power of more than 50 W. (See Fig. 15.)

Provided that the laser is used properly the protective measure of filters
and protective glasses recommended above are sufficient for avoiding accidents.
However, especially in case of endoscopic operations, it should be noted that
the laser beam should not be released until the laser endoscope has been inserted in the stomach or bladder or the organ in question.The opportunity for free
manipulation offered by the surgical handpiece necessitates special care and
demands the wearing of protective glasses in every case.

Based on the use and expertise established during the past five years, it
has proven that the proper application of the MediLas YAG laser, by adhering
to the pertinent safety precautions and a dosage which complies to the medical
indication, bears absolutely no risk on the safety of either patient or operating personnel.

REFERENCES

1. Kiefhaber, P., Nath, G., Moritz, K.: "Endoscopical Control of massive Gastrointestinal Hemorrhage by Irradiation with a High-Power Neodym-YAG Laser"
   Progr. Surg. 15 (1977), 140-155
2. Sander, P., Pösl, H., Spuhler, A., Hitzler, H.: "Der Neodym-YAG Laser: Ein
   effektives Instrument für die Stillung lebensbedrohlicher Gastrointestinal-
   blutungen" Leber Magen Darm 11 (1981), 31-36
3. Dierkesmann, R.: "Rekanalisation bronchialer Tumorstenosen mit dem Nd:YAG
   Laser" Internist 23 (1982), 283-286
4. Häußinger, K., Cujnik, F., Held, E., Heldwein, W., Zeiner, E.: "Bronchosko-
   pische Laserkoagulation zur Therapie des zentralen Bronchusverschlusses"
   Prax. Klin. Pneumol. 36 (1982), 471-474
5. Schlehe, H., Emslander, H.B., Weitprecht, M.: "Laserkoagulation mit dem
   Fibroskop" First. Meet. Deutsch. Ges. f. Lasermed., München, (1982)
6. Staehler, G., Hofstetter, A., Schmiedt, E., Keitisch, E., Gorisch, W.,
   Weinberg, W.: "Zerstörung von Blasentumoren durch endoskopische Laser-Bestrahlung" Deutsch. Ärzteblatt 75 (1978), 681-686
7. Hofstetter, A., Frank, F.: "Ein neues Laser-Endoskop zur Bestrahlung von
   Blasentumoren" Fortschr. Med. 97 (1979), 232-234
8. Staehler, G., Halldorsson, Th., Langerholc, J., Bilgram, R.: "Dosimetry for
   Neodym-YAG laser Applications in Urology" Laser Surg. and Med. 1 (1981)
   191-197
9. Hofstetter, A., Frank, F. et.al.: "The Neodym-YAG laser in Urology" Editions
   Roche, Basel, (1980)
10.Rothenberger, K., Pensel, J., Hofstetter, A., Keiditsch, E., Frank, F.:
   "Transurethral Laser Coagulation for Treatment of Urinary Bladder Tumors"
   Laser Surg. and Med. 2 (1983), 255-260
11.Hofstetter, A., Frank, F.: "The use of Lasers in Urology" in Surgical Applications of the Laser ed. Dixon, J.A. Year book Med. Pub., New York, (1983)
12.Perez-Castro Ellendt, E., Martinez-Pineiro, J.A.: "Transurethrale Uretero-
   pyeloskopie" Urologe A 20 (1981), 258-260
13.Hofstetter, A., Böwering, R., Keiditsch, E., Frank, F.: "Zerstörung von
   Uretertumoren mit dem Nd-YAG laser" Fortschr. Med. 101 (1983), 625-627
14.Beck, O.J.: "Comparative Studies on the Use of Lasers in Neurosurgery"
   MBB-AT Inform. 4/81 (1981)
15.Bailer, P.: "Tubensterilisation durch Laser-Koagulation" First. Meet.
   Deutsch. Ges. f. Lasermed., München, (1982)

16. Beck, O. J.: "The Use of the Nd-YAG and the CO_2 Laser in Neurosurgery" Neurosurg. Rev. 3 (1980), 261-266
17. Rothenberger, K., Hofstetter, A., Geiger, M., Böwering, R., Frank, F.: "Erfahrungsbericht über die externe Anwendung eines Neodym-YAG Lasers." Verhandlber. d. Deutsch. Ges. f. Uro. 31. Tag. (1979), 241-242
18. Staehler, G.: "Die externe Applikation von Neodym-YAG Laserstrahlen in der Urologie" Der Urologe A 20 (1981), 323-327
19. Landthaler, M., Haina, D., Waidelich, W., Braun-Falco, O.: "Therapeutische Laseranwendung in der Dermatologie" Der Hautarzt 32 (1981), 450-454
20. Frank, F., Halldorsson, Th., Manhardt, S., Kroy, W., Hofstetter, A., Pensel, J., Rothenberger, K.-H.: "Safety Aspects for Various Neodym-YAG Laser Applications".in Laser-Tokyo '81 ed. Atsumi, A. and Nimsakul, N. The Jap. Soc. f. Las. Med, Tokyo, (1981)

CHAPTER 24

THE BIOMEDICAL LASER: A MULTI-DISCIPLINARY

TOOL FOR THE 1980's

W.G. Solomon, President
Endo-Lase, Inc.
1729 21st Street, N.W.
Washington, D.C. 20009

THE BIOMEDICAL LASER:
A MULTI-DISCIPLINARY TOOL FOR THE 1980'S

W.G. Solomon, President
Endo-Lase, Inc., 1729 21st Street, N.W.
Washington, D.C. 20009

With several laser sources available in differing modes, each having its own biological effect on tissue, the choice of the physicican about which modality is appropriate for each specific purpose has not been well defined. The hospital administrator faced with conflicting laser requests from different services must first learn the physical principle of lasers and then master the complexities of the different wavelengths offered. He must select equipment which will fulfill the dual objective of improving patient care and of reducing the costs of hospitalization; but has a paucity of published information on which to base an informed decision.

We shall, therefore, be concerned here about the biological effects of lasers and in particular about the applicability and efficacy of the main laser types available. The most frequently used laser sources in medicine are Argon, Carbon Dioxide (CO_2) and Neodymium YAG (YAG) and their effectiveness is primarily determined by the absorption characteristics of the different wavelengths which they produce. It is the differentiated absorption in biological tissue which stimulates the various tissue effects which can be achieved.

THE ARGON LASER

Argon was the first laser to achieve general medical acceptance and this was in the field of Ophthalmology. Argon transmits a blue/green visible laser beam which can be transmitted through clear fluid. The wavelength (0.5 microns approximately) is selectively absorbed by pigmented tissue -- in the biological model specifically by hemaglobin and melanin. Small vessels can be readily coagulated by the precise Argon beam directed via the operating microscope, or the flexible fiber.

The Argon laser is a precise photocoagulator ideal for use on small diameter superficial blood vessels. It has found medical applications in the fields of Ophthalmology, Otology, Dermatology, Gastro-Enterology, Urology and Gynecology, and will be discussed further under each of these headings.

THE CARBON DIOXIDE LASER

The second laser to achieve significant medical acceptance was CO_2. This creates a beam of 10.6 microns which is in the mid inffa-red spectrum. Being invisible to the human eye, it is usually combined with a Helium-Neon (red) aiming beam. The CO_2 wavelength is specifically absorbed by water. As the human body is seventy to ninety percent water,

© 1983 by Elsevier Science Publishing Co., Inc.
Neodymium-YAG Laser in Medicine and Surgery, Joffe, Muckerheide, and Goldman, editors

the CO_2 laser is readily absorbed by the surface tissue. As a rule of thumb, the CO_2 laser is 90% absorbed within the first 1/10 mm. of tissue. The laser energy is converted into heat which instantaneously boils the cellular water, creating a vaporization crater. Owing to the very small spot size to which the beam can be focussed, this vaporization appears as a very precise cutting action. Vaporization of larger areas is best achieved by using the larger spot sizes available by alteration in the focus of the beam. The CO_2 laser is only a moderate coagulator. Focussed, it will seal blood vessels up to 0.5 mm. in diameter, and defocussed, with careful technique, vessels up to one mm. in diameter can be sealed. The major clinical applications for the CO_2 laser are in the fields of Neuro-Surgery, Gynecology, Laryngology, Plastic Surgery and Dermatology. At the present state of technology, the CO_2 laser can only be transmitted effectively via a mirrored articulated arm or micro-manipulator system.

THE NEODYMIUM YAG LASER

Most recently, the YAG laser has been gaining in medical acceptance. This laser produces a beam of 1.06 microns, in the near infra-red spectrum and being invisible to the human eye is, like the CO_2 laser, usually used in conjunction with a Helium-Neon (red) aiming beam.

The YAG wavelength is best absorbed by the color black. It is diffusely absorbed by body tissue thus permitting deep penetration of the laser energy. Heat builds up slowly allowing the operator to choose between coagulation and denaturation (low power and short exposures) or vaporization (high power and longer exposures). With the YAG laser, vessels of up to four or five mm. can be safely sealed. Once carbonization of tissue occurs, the absorption of the beam in the now blackened tissue allows the YAG laser to act as a cutting and vaporization instrument.

The YAG laser has its major applications in Gastro-enterology, Urology, Bronchology, Neurosurgery, Gynecology, Plastic Surgery and Dermatology.

A second and quite different YAG laser system is the Q-switched or mode locked version which produces high frequency pulses of very low wattage, but high peak power. The application of this equipment is limited to Ophthalmology.

The following chart will summarize the characteristics of the three laser types outlined, and it is their clinical applications which are of the greatest interest to practicing physicians and hospital administrators. It will be the purpose of the following section to discuss each wavelength within the context of the various subdisciplines which have adopted the bio-medical laser as a part of their armamentarium.

LASER MEDIUM	CO_2	ARGON	YAG
Type	Gas	Gas	Crystal
Wavelength	10.6 microns	0.5 microns	1.06 microns
Absorbed By	Water	Hemaglobin & Melanin	Tissue Protein
Penetration	1 mm.	2-3 mm.	5-7 mm.
Delivery	Mirror System	Fiber Optic	Fiber Optic
Coagulation	Low	Fair	High
Cutting	High	Low	Fair

OPHTHALMOLOGY

Ophthalmology was the first medical specialty to adopt the laser as an integral part of its standard surgical practice. The precise Argon beam directed via the slit lamp, passing through the aqueous and vitreous humors of the eye, is an ideal method for coagulating the small vessels which appear on the retina of diabetic patients. The technique has expanded to include other retinal vascularities and tears and has turned a traumatic operation requiring hospitalization and weeks of recuperation into a virtually painless outpatient procedure -- frequently carried out in the doctor's office.

After many cataract procedures, especially those using the extra-capsulary technique, the posterior membrane of the eye clouds over. Conventionally, this is treated by slitting the membrane with a scalpel. A new method of using the low power, but high frequency pulsed YAG laser (Q-switched or mode locked) shatters this with a shock wave effect. This has become the most demanded technique by Ophthalmologists today.

The treatment of Glaucoma has been carried out with some success both by Argon and YAG lasers, and this technique is expected to develop in popularity with the availability of a new generation of ophthalmic YAG lasers. The CO_2 laser has been used experimentally for corneal tumors, but up to now this application has had no general acceptance.

OTOLARYNGOLOGY

The CO_2 laser has won wide acceptance in this specialty for its ability to vaporize papillomata of the vocal chords. These are removed under precise microscopic control with minimal trauma to the chords and excellent re-epithelialization of the tissue. Small tumors have also been treated by this method, as have a wide variety of oral lesions such as leukoplakia and hemangiomata.

The Argon laser has a special place in the surgical removal of stapes footplate.

The YAG laser has been used for its superior coagulative properties in oral surgery -- especially in the treatment of hemophiliacs. Vocal chord polyps and tumors may also be treated by YAG and deep seated hemangiomata are best treated by YAG, as there is no cratering effect.

It may be helpful to use the vocal chord polyp as an example of the quite different tissue effects of the CO_2 and YAG lasers.

The CO_2 laser vaporizes the polyp by boiling the cell water. The polyp literally disappears in smoke and leaves a small crater which rapidly heals over.

The YAG laser denaturates the polyp at a lower, non boiling temperature. The supply blood vessels are occluded and the polyp turns white. It may be plucked off or left to slough off and either way leaves a dry bed which rapidly heals over.

GASTRO-ENTEROLOGY

The YAG laser used in conjunction with the fiber optic gastroscope provides an opportunity to turn diagnostic endoscopy into a therapeutic procedure. All types of bleeding in the gastro-intestinal tract can be stopped. Smaller lesions will be permanently sealed, although a high proportion of esophageal varices will re-bleed at a later date. Emergency surgery can be prevented, allowing the surgical procedure to take place on a stabilized patient in a planned manner. It has been demonstrated that this decreases the high mortality rates associated with emergency surgery on acutely bleeding patients.

The only difference between internal and external bleeding is one of access. The patient bleeding acutely from external injury always has his bleeding controlled mechanically on entry to the emergency room. The YAG laser brings the potential of treating emergency internal bleeding via a laser hemostat -- saving the patient the risks and costs associated with multi-unit blood transfusions.

The Argon laser has also been used for the control of gastro-intestinal bleeding. It is effective in coagulating small more superficial vessels and it was for a time considered to be safer in use, owing to its lower depth of penetration. Experience has shown that perforation with the YAG laser has been a very rare occurrence. The history of laser use in the discipline shows that Argon users have nearly all added YAG to their armamentarium in order to expand their capabilities.

Obstructive tumors of the esophagus are now being treated by YAG laser. This palliative treatment first coagulates the tumor, denaturing it by sealing the internal blood vessels. At higher powers, the laser vaporizes the necrotic mass, which can also be removed mechanically by grasping forceps. A new lumen is created through which the patient can swallow, dramatically improving the quality and in some cases length of life. The initial studies have been successful and carried out with minimal complications. A similar procedure is being used for palliation of obstructive tumors of the colon and rectum.

The CO_2 laser has found no applications so far in the field of Gastro-Enterology.

UROLOGY

The treatment of bladder tumors has proved an important area for the YAG laser. The YAG laser can be added to the standard modus operandi of the Urologist and, using a modified Alberran bridge, all areas of the bladder can be reached. The use of the laser reduces localized recurrences and makes the use of the post operative indwelling catheter unnecessary. There is experimental evidence that lymphatics are sealed, preventing interoperative spread of malignancy. Patients may return home sooner, frequently on the same day, and the requirement for follow-up procedures is reduced. The savings in cost are clear.

Tumors of the lower ureter can be treated with an adapted ureterscope. New techniques are proving successful in the treatment of urethral strictures and condylomata accuminata are effectively destroyed. Some cases of penile carcinoma have been treated, and there is hope that YAG laser will prove a safe alternative to amputation.

The Argon laser has been used with some success for Arterio-Venus malformations of the bladder, but does not have sufficient penetrative power to photocoagulate bladder tumors.

The CO_2 laser is absorbed by water, so that its use would require the Urologist to change technique and operate in a gas filled bladder. It would vaporize surface tumors, but without providing the full thickness coagulation necrosis effected by the YAG laser. The CO_2 laser deals effectively with condylomata and other lesions of the external genitalia.

GYNECOLOGY

The treatment of cervical intra-epithelial neoplasia by CO_2 laser is a well accepted and effective technique. Under microscopic control, the cervix can be vaporized down to the depth desired by the Gynecologist. The new micro-scanning techniques increase the accuracy of this procedure. Laser treatment can be given on an outpatient basis and where cone biopsy is the preferred treatment, the use of the CO_2 laser increases accuracy and reduces blood loss. The CO_2 laser is effective in the treatment of condylomata accuminata and some investigators are reporting success in reducing recurrences of acute herpes after laser vaporization.

Recently, the CO_2 laser has found an important application in the lysis of adhesions. The precise cutting action in conjunction with the hemostatic properties of the CO_2 laser seems to prevent adhesion reformation. In tubal re-anastamosis, the CO_2 laser provides a clean cut and dry fallopian tube edge for suturing. Good pregnancy figures have been reported.

The Argon laser, because of its selective absorption in blood, is being used in the treatment of endometriosis.

The special place of the YAG laser in Gynecology is for the photovaporization of the endometrium as an alternative to hysterectomy in cases of non-malignant dysfunctional bleeding. A major surgical intervention is changed into an outpatient procedure with obvious benefits to the patient -- reduction of trauma, saving in cost and the elimination of time away from work. The YAG laser is an effective method for laparascopic sterilization. By sealing the fallopian tubes with less tissue destruction than by the conventional bi-polar coagulation there should be an improved success with subsequent reversal procedures. Pelvic endometriosis is also effectively treated through the laparascope. The YAG laser will denaturate condylomata and may also be used in the treatment of cervical neoplasia with good depth of penetration and sealing of lymphatics.

NEUROSURGERY

The precise nature of laser surgery has made Neurosurgeons particularly interested in the use of the laser. The CO_2 laser has won acceptance for its precise dissection of healthy brain tissue and its ability to vaporize tumors without trauma to adjacent vital structures. Acoustic and spinal tumors have been treated as well as intra-cranial malignancies. The post operative recovery is enhanced by the non-touch technique and reduction in thermal damage.

The YAG laser has been used in Neurosurgery over the same period of time, but in many fewer centers. The specific indications for YAG are vascular tumors (meningiomas and A.V.M.'s), sinus invasive tumors and intra-ventricular tumors. Its superior coagulative effect has proved of benefit in the treatment of some highly vascular conditions with considerable savings in operating time and with excellent post-operative results. The fiber optic delivery system presents the opportunity for endoscopic laser neurosurgery. Using the YAG laser to photo-coagulate the tumor bed has been effective in reducing local recurrences.

The Argon laser has also been used in Neurosurgery and its extremely small spot size in conjunction with its coagulation properties has given it limited applications in this field.

There seems little doubt but that Neurosurgeons will turn in increasing numbers to laser surgery, especially now that the precision of lasers is combined with the coagulation properties of the YAG wavelength.

PULMONARY MEDICINE/THORACIC SURGERY

The palliative treatment of obstructing endobronchial tumors by YAG laser has attracted much interest over the past two years. These tumors can be denatured and photo-coagulated and the necrotic material is removed by grasping forceps. A new lumen is created and patients can breathe. Some dramatic clinical results have been obtained and X-rays demonstrate reventilation of previously occluded lungs. The technique can be carried out either using local anesthesia and flexible bronchoscopy or general anesthesia and the rigid bronchoscope. Using a similar technique, trachial stenoses may also be treated.

The CO_2 laser has some application through specially adapted laser bronchoscopes. It cannot be used on vascular tumors, as the coagulative powers are not sufficient to stop bleeding in this inaccessible area.

The Argon laser is being used as an energy source for a Dye Laser in the treatment of early, non-invasive bronchial tumors. The patient is injected with Hematoporphyrin Derivative -- a dye which remains in the tumor cell after it has migrated from healthy tissue. This is photo-sensitized by the wavelength [6.30 microns] from the Rhodamine dye. The technique is effective for early non-invasive endo-bronchial tumors, but cannot be used on obstructive tumors, as it is not possible to control penetration depths and perforation risks are therefore unacceptable.

PLASTIC SURGERY AND DEMATOLOGY

The treatment of all kinds of skin lesions and soft tissue tumors has been undertaken by all three laser types. From Port Wine Stains, to the removal of tattoos, from superficial telangectasia to cavernous hemangiomata, from plantar warts to varicose veins, from melanoma to keratosis -- all have been treated and described in the literature by CO_2, Argon and YAG. The only clear guideline is that there is as yet no concensus as to which modality works best in any given clinical condition.

It may be helpful, therefore, to go back to first principles. Where excision is required, the CO_2 laser will be the modality of choice; where small blood vessels need coagulation, the Argon would be preferred; where deep seated lesions are encountered, the YAG would be the most effective. The Dermatologist can be assured that whichever laser type is purchased by his hospital, he will be able to utilize it to treat a wide variety of the conditions which he encounters among his patients.

GENERAL SURGERY

In spite of repeated attempts to interest general surgeons in laser surgery, no modality has yet won wide acceptance. There are, however, many procedures in which lasers can be of benefit. Broadly, they are useful in operating through infected tissue and in achieving hemostasis -- areas where the electro cautery unit is either ineffective or too damaging. Lasers will win increasing acceptance for use in the debulking of large vascular tumors (YAG), for kidney bivalve procedures to remove staghorn calculi (CO_2), for partial splenectomies (YAG), for liver resection (YAG), for Mastectomies, especially with fungating tumors (CO_2), for hemorrhoidectomies (CO_2 and YAG), for debriding decubitus ulcers (CO_2 and YAG), in Burn Surgery (CO_2 and YAG).

RESEARCH AREAS

There are two disciplines in which research into laser applications is extremely active, but which have not yet reached the clinical stage. In Orthopedic Surgery, there is eager anticipation of the Laser Menisectomy through the Arthroscope. There is also some reason to believe that the application of lasers to arthritic joints may provide some relief and remission. In Cardiology, it is believed that the laser may be used to remove plaques from sclerotic arteries. The technique is successful experimentally, but the delivery of the laser energy in an acceptable multi-core cannula needs further miniaturization. Animal hearts have been revascularized and small blood vessels have been re-anastamosed. The Cardiovascular applications of lasers are only now being developed, but there is much promise in the experimental work being undertaken in many different laboratories.

It will be apparent from the above that the use of the bio-medical laser in the hospital has already moved away from the early pioneering situation to one of everyday clinical use and acceptance. Hospitals will in the near future have not just one laser, but the whole range of wavelengths available. The development will be speeded up by the growth in laser training courses which educate physicians in ever increasing numbers and the growing realization that laser surgery reduces hospital costs and is of significant assistance to administrators in their constant efforts toward the containment of hospital costs.

224

ACKNOWLEDGEMENTS

A bibliography to cover so many disciplines and laser
types would be longer than the chapter, and I hope to be
forgiven for its omission. I would instead like to thank the
many physicians both in the United States and in Europe who
have taken the time to teach me about laser applications in
their field. In particular, I would thank Isaac Kaplan, who
first interested me in surgical lasers and spent hours passing
on to me his voluminous knowledge; Malcolm Anderson and Albert
Singer taught me the little I know of Gynecology, and Milton
Goldrath has recently augmented this by explaining his
procedure for endometrial photo-coagulation. In Neurosurgery
Peter Ascher has been my teacher, and in Gastroenterology I
am indebted first to Stephen Joffe and then to Richard Dwyer,
who has such enthusiasm for and knowledge of applications in
this and so many other areas. In Urology, Professor Hofstetter
is pre-eminent in the laser field, and I was privileged to
spend time with him. In Dermatology, Philip Bailin has been
most informative about the use of the different wavelengths.
In Bronchoscopy, Michael Unger has been one of the pioneers
in the United States and has freely shared his knowledge and
enthusiasm. In Orthopedics, Dick Caspari explained his
innovative ideas to me, and in General Surgery, Harvey White
has been willing to use the laser in a variety of interesting
procedures. Kenneth Fox has outlined to me the many uses of
the laser in Ophthalmology. In all these disciplines and for
his thoughtful advice in so many ways, I shall always remain
indebted to John Dixon, who has an incomparable experience
and knowledge of all these applications of the biomedical
laser.

None of the above are in any way responsible for the
contents of this chapter, but they have over the years given
me the specialist knowledge which has made this overview a
possibility.

CHAPTER 25

CURRENT STATUS OF THE Nd:YAG MEDICAL LASER

(A Multidisciplinary Device)

Principal Author:

Anthony A. Goossens
Molectron Medical
Sunnyvale, California

CURRENT STATUS OF THE Nd:YAG MEDICAL LASER
(A Multidisciplinary Device)

Anthony A. Goossens, Charles E. Enderby, Ph.D., Sandra Gilbert
Molectron Medical, Sunnyvale, California

The Nd:YAG laser had its beginning during the early sixties.
It was not until the mid-1970's, with the work of Fruhmorgen (1)
and Kiefhaber (2) that this device was applied to clinical
studies. Since those early years the Nd:YAG laser has been used
extensively in the field of medical therapy.

THE BASIC Nd:YAG LASER

The Nd:YAG, a solid state laser, is a relatively simple device as represented in Figure 1.

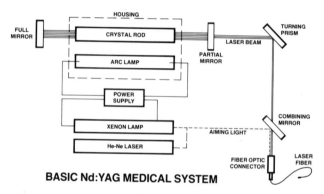

BASIC Nd:YAG MEDICAL SYSTEM

Figure 1. The components of a Nd:YAG Laser

At the heart of this laser lies a crystalline rod. This rod
is grown by combining yttrium, aluminum and garnet (YAG) and
doping it with a few percent of neodymium (Nd) ions. It is about
10 cm long and 6 mm in diameter and can be made to lase by
supplying energy from a powerful arc lamp (5000 watts). Both
the lamp and crystalline rod are enclosed within a gold coated
housing. The gold coat acts as a reflector to increase the
energy pumped into the rod, which increases the population inversion of the electrons. Photons are produced with this population inversion. Most of the photons created, about 97%, are
lost as heat. A small portion of the emission travels to the
mirrors at each end of the rod, is reflected through the rod and
is coherently amplified. Of the two mirrors, only one is 100%
reflector while the other is a partial reflector. Once the laser
beam is formed, it can exit through the partial reflector and is
coupled into a fiber optic.

The Nd:YAG laser operates in the infrared region, 1060 nm, and
is invisible to the human eye. A xenon lamp, which produces a
bright white light, is used as an aiming light. White light is
highly visible on blood or reddish tissue. On white tissue,
such as found in the central nervous system, a He-Ne laser is
used to produce a red light. Either of the two aiming lights,
xenon or He-Ne, can be used to direct the Nd:YAG laser beam.

© 1983 by Elsevier Science Publishing Co., Inc.
Neodymium-YAG Laser in Medicine and Surgery, Joffe, Muckerheide, and Goldman, editors

FIBER OPTICS

As laser technology progresses, dramatic changes will take place in fiber optics and other attachments. The basic laser will show little change, due to the physics of the device.

Present fiber delivery systems are composed of fibers with a quartz core surrounded by a silicone rubber cladding and a teflon cover. The quartz core, cladding and teflon cover are enclosed with a polyethylene catheter, Figure 2. The fiber is encased in a catheter which provides protection to the fiber and permits gas or water to flow between the fiber and catheter to clear the treatment site. Fibers may range from 50 μm to 1000μm in diameter. The divergence angle of the laser beam at the tip of the catheter is typically between 8 to 12 degrees. These fibers are very flexible and can be used in conjunction with endoscopes, or attached to microscopes or hand pieces for focussed applications.

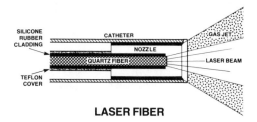

LASER FIBER

Figure 2. Composition of a typical fiber delivery system

The flexible quartz fiber and its catheter are easily inserted into most endoscopes. Scope manufacturers such as Olympus, Fujinon, Pentax, ACMI, etc., provide scopes with biopsy channels ranging from 1.2 mm to 5.0 mm. The laser system couples to fibers for most of these scopes and are easily interchanged.

Fibers can be passed down the endoscope and extended to the treatment site. Once the fiber is visible, just beyond the scope, it is brought to within 1-2 cm of the site. This appears to be the normal distance for laser application. Since there is no tissue contact, the possibility of infection is reduced. The laser is fired, via a foot switch, and has the ability to coagulate or vaporize tissue depending on the power setting or the exposure time.

THE INSTRUMENT

The Nd:YAG laser, Figure 3, is composed of a variety of delicate optics which require critical alignments. When the laser beam emerges from its source, it is approximately 6 mm in diameter. The beam must be focussed to enter a fiber coupler that has a diameter of 0.6 mm. The white or red aiming light must also enter this fiber attachment.

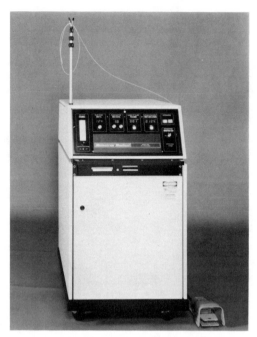

Figure 3.   Molectron Model 8000 Nd:YAG Laser

Lasers are sensitive to temperature changes and vibrations. To prevent the optics from shifting out of alignment, they are mounted on a kinematic deck which is impervious to radical temperature changes or strong vibrations.

The laser must be adaptable and mobile to be used as a multi-disciplinary device.   To be adaptable, it requires a wide range of power outputs, different delivery systems fibers, hand pieces and microscope attachments.   Mobility requires shock mounted optics, low center of gravity so it cannot tip over, large casters to cross over obstructions such as elevator gaps, and quick disconnects on the cooling hoses.

All Nd:YAG lasers must be calibrated periodically.   Calibration should be a quick and simple built-in procedure where the actual laser output can be measured.

The Nd:YAG laser is a relatively easy instrument to operate, requiring no special electrical or mechanical engineering skills. There are only a few controls that need to be preset: 1) number of watts, 2) exposure time, 3) gas flow.

The foot switch activates the laser and is limited to the exposure time set on the console.   If the foot switch is released early the laser will cease to fire.

BIOLOGICAL INTERACTION

When a laser beam is directed at tissues, a thermal or photo reaction occurs. It's absorption by the tissue will vary with its optical characteristics. The more opaque or pigmented tissues are, the more energy that will be absorbed (3).

Several factors influence absorption levels of laser energy, Figure 4 illustrates a few of these factors.

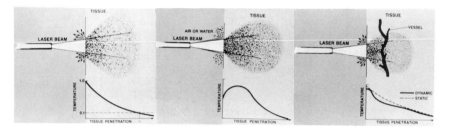

static   dynamic   dynamic

Figure 4.   Tissue penetration vs. temperature when
            comparing static and dynamic systems

In a static system, the tissue is uniform and the laser beam penetrates a homogeneous environment. This is rarely, if ever, the case. Tissue being treated may be cooled with air or water, is not perfectly smooth, does not remain stationary, and is not homogeneous due to vascularity and other factors. Considerations such as power density of the laser beam, exposure time and surface tensions must also be considered.

When laser energy enters the tissue it is both scattered and absorbed. This absorption determines the axial penetration, while scattering determines the zone around the axis. Both can be measured by the thermal energy or heat. This heat, which interacts with tissue is the main mechanism for therapy and/or destruction. When tissue absorbs heat and reaches approximately 42°C, denaturation of protein or thermal coagulation occurs. Cell death often results from coagulation and can be therapeutic if necrosis results in cessation of bleeding and regeneration of viable tissue (4).

At temperatures greater than 42°C, veins and arteries begin to shrink and eventually vaporize. These reactions may take place in a short time, less than a second, depending on the power output of the laser.

The Nd:YAG laser beam has low surface absorption and penetrates tissue to a depth of 4.0 mm. Penetration depth is

defined as the amount of energy that passes through tissue and
reaches a point where the intensity falls to 10% of the initial
value. Power output of the laser system can exceed 120 watts,
which is enough energy to overcome the dynamic conditions of
tissue. This will permit deep thermal coagulation, tissue
destruction and tumor removal.

CURRENT APPLICATIONS

The Nd:YAG laser is currently being investigated in various
disciplines, such as Gastroenterology; Pulmonary/Bronchoscopy;
Urology; Neurosurgery; Gynecology; Dermatology; Cardiology; and
Orthopedics. Each of these disciplines will be briefly discussed citing several clinical investigators who have written
extensive articles in each field.

GASTROINTESTINAL APPLICATIONS

Initial investigations of the Nd:YAG laser were conducted
by gastroenterologists. During the past decade many investigators have treated numerous patients. These treatments have
included: 1) Ablation of esophageal obstructions or tumors,
2) ablation of colonic tumors, 3) treatment of non-bleeding
angiodysplasia, and 4) coagulation of bleeding from: ulcers,
Mallory-Weiss tears, esophageal varcies, angiodysplasia.

Several clinical investigators who are using the Nd:YAG
laser have published articles describing their findings:
Brunetaud(7), Bown (5,6), Cummins (8), Dixon (9,10,11), Fleischer
(12,13,14,15,16), Ichikawa (17), Ito (18), Iwaski (19), Johnston
(20,21), Halldorsson (22, 23), and Silverstein (24,25).

By the first half of this year, 1983, there were an estimated 200 centers worldwide, using the Nd:YAG laser for various
applications. At least half of the centers were using the laser
for gastrointestinal therapy.

UROLOGICAL APPLICATIONS

In recent years, urological applications of Nd:YAG lasers
have attracted clinical investigators. A variety of patients
with different conditions have been treated. Treatments have included: 1) Destruction of malignant lesions of the bladder wall,
2) destruction of benign lesions, 3) coagulation of vascularities of the bladder wall, and 4) albation of: urethral tumors,
ureter tumors, condylomata accuminata, carcinoma of the penis.

Several clinical investigators have published articles describing their findings. A sample of investigators are: Bulow
(26,27,28), Hofstetter (29,20,31,32), Keiditsch (33,34), McPhee
(35,36,37), Staehler (38,39,40), Frank (42,43), Pensel (44), and
Dixon (45).

PULMONARY/THORACIC APPLICATIONS

Another recent application of the Nd:YAG laser has been
Pulmonary/Thoracic therapy. Treatments have included: 1) destruction of stenosis after tracheostomy or surgery, 2) destruction of granulomas (chondroma and adenoma), 3) coagulation of
bleeding lesions, 4) relief of dyspnea, 5) ablation of

atelectasis or obstructive pneumonites.

Clinical investigators who have published articles describing their findings are: Cortese (46), Dixon (47), Dumon (48,49, 50), Jain (51,52), McDougall (53), Nagasawa (54), Oho (55), Ohtani (56), Personne (57), Tamada (58), Toty (59,60), Vourc'h (61), and Yamada (62).

NEUROSURGERY APPLICATIONS

Neurosurgery with the laser has been conducted mainly with the CO_2 laser. Some recent applications with the Nd:YAG have been: 1) Resection of cerebral arteriovenous malformations, 2) ablation of: meningiomas and hermengiomas, 3) sinus invasive tumors, 4) intraventricular tumors, and 5) pituitary tumors.

Clinical investigators who have published articles include: Saunders (63), and Taki (64).

OBSTETRICS/GYNECOLOGY APPLICATIONS

Obstetrics and Gynecology is still a new area of research as far as the Nd:YAG laser is concerned. Most laser studies have been conducted with the CO_2 laser. There are some direct applications where the Nd:YAG laser has had some affect. Treatments have included: 1) Coagulation of endometriosis, 2) opening of ovarian cysts, 3) coagulation during tumor resection, 4) palliation of Paget's disease of the vulva, 5) removal of condylomata acuminata, and 6) vaporization of the endometrium for the treatment of menorrhagia.

Goldrath (65) published an article describing the use of the Nd:YAG laser on photovaporization of endometrium for the treatment of menorrhagia.

DERMATOLOGY/CANCER APPLICATIONS

In dermatology and skin cancer the Nd:YAG has only limited applications. The Argon laser has been more effective in this area. The Nd:YAG has been investigated for the following applications: 1) Ablation of skin tumors, 2) removal of keloids, 3) lightening of tatoos.

Clinical investigators who have published articles describing their findings include: 1) Kozlov (66), Lee (67), and Noe (68).

CARDIOLOGY AND ORTHOPEDIC APPLICATIONS

Some preliminary work has been done with the Nd:YAG to vaporize atheromas in arteries. In the heart, myocardial revascularization has been attempted by drilling holes in the myocardium (69). for orthopedics the laser has been investigated for removal of torn meniscus.

LASER SAFETY

Precautions must be takne when using the Nd:YAG laser by both the operating room personnel and the patient. These precautions must consider ophthalmic and skin exposures. A laser beam striking the eye may cause considerable damage, depending upon its intensity. Reflective light may have enough energy to cause injuries.

Most structures of the eye can be damaged, but the retina is the most sensitive. In particular, the pigment epithelium could be destroyed and would not regenerate in its original light-sensitive form; this would result in lost vision (70).

Safe levels of ophthalmic exposure to laser energy have been established by the American National Standard, Table 1.

OPHTHALMIC SAFETY

ANS SAFE LEVEL IS 8mW/cm² AT CORNEA OF EYE

ENDOSCOPIC SYSTEM 100 – 200mW/cm²
FILTER BY 1000 TO 0.1 TO 0.2mW/cm²

OPEN SYSTEM 10,000mW/cm² (100W at 25cm)
FILTER BY 4500 TO 6000 TO < 2mW/cm²

Table 1: Ophthalmic Safety standards

Studies (71) have shown that for typical treatment levels of Nd:YAG laser, the reflected light from the mucosa up through the endoscope can be in the order of 100 to 200 mW/cm², thereby requiring the use of a filter over the ocular of the endoscope. The ocular filter attentuates laser energy to about 1,000 resulting in reflective light well below the hazardous level.

Laser exposure to the skin is less hazardous than ophthalmic exposure, and usually does not cause permanent damage. Effects from accidental exposures vary from mild reddening to blisters and charring (72).

FUTURE OF THE Nd:YAG Laser

Nd:YAG laser therapy is just emerging from its pioneering stage. The laser's ability to coagulate and vaporize tissue has increased its potential in many medical applications. Thousands of patients have been treated to date, and preliminary data suggest positive benefits. In the future the Nd:YAG laser could play a vital role in the treatment of medical disorders.

BIBLIOGRAPHY

1. Fruhmorgen P, Reidenbach J, Bodem R, Demling L:
   Experimental Examination on Laser Endoscopy. Endoscopy
   6:116, 1974.

2. Kiefhaber P, Nath G, Moritz K: Endoscopic Control of Massive
   Gastrointestinal Hemorrhage by Irradiation With a High-power
   Nd:YAG laser. Progress in Surgery 15:140, 1977.

3. Hillenkamp F. (1979) Interaction Between Laser Radiation and
   Biological Systems. Lasers In Biology and Medicine. Plenum
   Press, New York pp37-68.

4. Goossens A, Enderby C: Fundamentals of Medical Lasers.
   Gastrointestinal Endoscopy (in press 1983).

5. Bown S, Salmon P, Kelly D, Calder B, Pearson H, Weaver B:
   Nd:YAG Laser Photocoagulation in the Dog Stomach and a
   Comparison With Argon Laser Results. Presented at the Int'l
   Medical Laser Symposium. Detroit, March 1979.

6. Bown S, Salmon P, Storey D, Calder B, Kelly D, Adams N,
   Pearson H, Weaver B: Nd:YAG Laser Photocoagulation in the
   Dog Stomach. Journal of the British Society of Gastro-
   enterology GUT, 21:818, 1980.

7. Bruentaud J, Houcke P, DeMotte J, Mosquet T, Paris J: Laser
   in Digestive Endoscopy. Abst. pres. at the 4th Congress of
   Int'l Society for Laser Surgery. Tokyo, 20:31, 1981.

8. Cummins L: Laser-tissue Interaction. Proc. of Therapeutic
   Laser Endoscopy. Chicago, 1982.

9. Dixon J, Berenson M, McCloskey D: Nd:YAG Laser Treatment of
   Experimental Canine Gastric Bleeding. Gastroenterology,
   77:4(1):647-651, 1979.

10. Dixon J: Endoscopic Laser Surgery: Narrow Focus but
    Numerous Targets. Medical News, 245(16):1623 4/24/81.

11. Dixon J. (1983) Surgical Application of Lasers. Year Book
    Medical Publishers, Inc. 204pgs.

12. Fleischer D: Gastrointestinal Laser Activity in the U.S.
    Presented at the 13th Int'l Congress on Stomach Disease.
    Antwerp, May 1981.

13. Fleischer D: Palliative Therapy for Esophageal Carcinoma by
    Endoscopic Nd:YAG Laser. Abstracts pres. at the 4th Congress
    of Int'l Society for Laser Surgery. Tokyo, 20:17 1981.

14. Fleischer D, Kessler F, Haye O: Endoscopic Nd:YAG Laser
    Therapy for Carcinoma of the Esophagus: A New Palliative
    Approach.   The American Journal of Surgery, 143:280 1982.

15. Fleischer D: The Current Status of Gastrointestinal Laser
    Activity in the United States.   Gastrointestinal Endoscopy,
    28(3):157, 1982.

16. Fleischer D: Endoscopic Laser Therapy for Upper Gastro-
    intestinal Tract Disease.   Surv. Dig. Dis. 1:42-53, 1983.

17. Ichikawa T, Nakasawa S, Ema Y: Effects of Nd:YAG Laser
    Irradiation on the Gastric Cancers, Including Histology.
    Abst. Pres. at the 4th Congress of Int'l Society for Laser
    Surgery.   Tokyo, 5:18-21, 1981.

18. Ito Y, Sugiura H, Kano T, Kiraoka Y, Kasugai T: Endoscopic
    Laser Treatment of Borderline Lesions and Early Gastric
    Carcinoma.   Abst. pres. at the 4th Congress of Int'l Society
    of Laser Surgery.   Tokyo, 20:10-12, 1981.

19. Iwasaki, M, Sasako M, Konishi T, Maruyama Y, Wada T:
    Clinical Applications of the Nd:YAG Endoscopy.   Abst. Pres.
    at the 4th Congress of Int'l Society for Laser Surgery.
    Tokyo, 5:14-17, 1981.

20. Johnston J, Jensen D, Mautner W, Elashoff J: YAG Laser
    Treatment of Experimental Bleeding Canine Gastric Ulcers.
    Gastroenterology, 79:1252-1261, 1980.

21. Johnston J, Jensen D, Mautner W: Comparison of Endoscopic
    Electrocoagulation & Laser Photocoagulation of Bleeding
    Canine Bastric Ulcers.   Gastroenterology, 82:904, 1982.

22. Halldorsson T, Langerholc J: Thermodynamic Analysis of Laser
    Irradiation of Biological Tissue.   Applied Optics.
    17(24):3948, 1978.

23. Halldorsson T, Rother W, Langerholc J, Frank F: Theoretical
    and Experimental Investigations Prove Nd:YAG Laser Treatment
    to be Safe.   Presented at the Int'l Medical Laser Symposium.
    Detroit, March 1979.

24. Silverstein F: Round Table Discussion on Control of
    Gastrointestinal Bleeding.   Int'l Symposium on Digestive
    Endoscopy.   Paris, Oct. 1978.

25. Silverstein F, Protell R, Gilbert D, Gulacsik C, Auth D,
    Dennis M, Rubin C: Argon vs. Nd:YAG Laser Photocoagulation
    of Experimental Canine Bastric Ulcers.   Gastroenterology.
    77:491-496, 1979.

26. Bulow H, Bulow U, Frohmuller H: Laser Investigations of the Strictured Dog Urethra, Investigative Urology, 16(5):403, 1978.

27. Bulow H: Present Status of Endoscopic Laser Treatments in Urology. Endoscopy, 4:240, 1979.

28. Bulow H, Bulow U, Frohmuller H: Transurethral Laser Urethotomy in Man. The Journal of Urology, 121:286, 1979.

29. Hofstetter A, Rothenberger K, Keiditsch E, Frank F, Pensel J, Bowering R, Henneberger G: The Efficiency of the Nd:YAG Laser in Urinary Bladder Treatment. Abst. of pres. at the 4th Congress of the Int'l Society for Laser Surgery. Tokyo, 10:18, 1981.

30. Hofstetter A, Staehler G, Keiditsch E, Frank F: Laser Treatment of Carcinoma of the Penis. Journal of Medicine, 96(8):369-371, 1978.

31. Hofstetter A, Frank F: The Neodymium-YAG Laser in Urology. Editiones "Roche," F. Hoffman-LaRoche & Co., Ltd., Basel, Switzerland, 1980.

32. Hofstetter A, Frank F: A New Laser Endoscope for the Treatment of Tumors of the Bladder. Fortschritte der Medizin, 97(6) Feb 5, 1979.

33. Keiditsch E, Stern J, Zimmerman I, Hofstetter A, Frank F, Pensel J, Rothenberger K: Interruption of Urinary Bladder Wall Lymph Drainage by Nd:YAG Laser Irradiation. Abst. of pres. at the 4th Congress of the Int'l Society for Laser Surgery; Tokyo, 10:48, 1981.

34. Keiditsch E, Hofstetter A, Rothenberger K, Maiwald H, Stern J, Pensel J, Frank F: Comparative Morphological Investigations of the Effects of Neodymium-YAG Laser and Electro-coagulation In Experimental Animal Research. Int'l Congress on Gynecologic Laser Surgery. New Orleans, LA Jan. 9-12, 1980.

35. Segmental Irradiation of the Bladder with a Nd:YAG Laser Resectoscope. Abst. of pres. at the 4th Congress of the Int'l Society for Laser Surgery. Tokyo, 10:42, 1981.

36. Laser Resectoscope Preliminary Animal Investigations. Abst. of pres. at the 4th Congress of Int'l Society for Laser Surgery. Tokyo, 17:31, 1981.

37. Segmental Irradiation of the Bladder with Neodymium YAG Laser Irradiation. Journal of Urology, 128:1101, 1982.

236

38. Dosimetry for Neodymium:YAG Laser Applications for Urology. Presented at the Int'l Medical Laser Symposium. Detroit, March 29,-31, 1979.

39. Staehler G, McCord R, Hofstetter A, Keiditsch R: Nd:YAG Laser Irradiation of the Normal and Tumorous Bladder Wall. Presented at the 2nd International Symposium on Laser Surgery. Texas. Oct. 23-26, 1977.

40. Staehler G, Kronester A, Weinberg W, Keiditsch E, McCord R, Hofstetter A: Thermal Damage to the Intestine by Nd:YAG Laser Application to the Bladder. Presented at the Int'l Congress on Laser Surgery. New Orleans, LA Jan. 1980.

41. Staehler G, Haldorsson T, Langerholc J, Bilgram R: Dosimetry for Nd:YAG Laser Applications in Urology. Lasers in Surgery And Medicine, 1(2):191-197, 1980.

42. Frank F, Hofstetter A, Keiditsch E: Experimental Investigation and New Instrumentation for Nd:YAG Laser Treatment in Urology. Int'l Congress on Gynecologic Laser Surgery. New Orleans, LA Jan. 9-12, 1980.

43. Frank F, Keiditsch E, Hofstetter A, Pensel J, Rothenberger K: Various Effects of the CO_2, the Neodymium-YAG and the Argon Laser Irradiation on Bladder Tissue. Lasers in Surgery and Medicine, 2:89-96, 1982.

44. Pensel J, Frank F, Rothenberger K, Hofstetter A, Unsold E: Destruction of Urinary Calculi by Neodymium-YAG Laser Irradiation. Abst. of Pres. at the 4th Congress of Int'l Society for Laser Surgery, Tokyo, 10:4, 1981.

45. Dixon J. (1983) Surgical Application of Lasers. Year Book Medical Publishers, Inc. 204 pgs.

46. Cortese D, Kinsey J: Endoscopic Management of Lung Cancer With Hematoporphyrin Derivative Phototherapy. Mayo Clinic Proc. 57:543-47, 1982.

47. Dixon J. (1983) Surgical Application Of Lasers. Year Book Medical Publishers, Inc. 204 pgs.

48. Dumon J, Meric B, Velardocchio J, Garbe L, Saux P: YAG Laser Resection of Trachea Bronchial Lesions. Abst. from 4th Congr. of Int'l Society for Laser Surgery, Tokyo. 14:28-31, 1981.

49. Dumon J, Reboud, Garbe L, Aucomte F, Meric B: Treatment of Tracheobronchial Lesions by Laser Photoresection. Chest, 81(3):278 1982.

50. Dumon J, Bourcereau J, Meric B, Aucomte F, Dupin B: Report
    of 1000 YAG Laser Endobronchial Resections.   Presented at the
    Annual Meeting of the American Thoracic Society, Kansas City,
    May, 1983.

51. Jain K, Gorisch W: Microvascular Repair with Neodymium-YAG
    Laser. Acta Neurochir (Wien) 28:260-262,1979.

52. Jain K: Sutureless Microvascular Anastomosis Using A
    Neodymium-YAG Laser.   Journal of Microsurgery, 1:436-439,
    1980.

53. McDougall J, Cortese D: Neodymium YAG Laser Therapy of Mal-
    ignant Airway Obstruction.   Mayo Clinic Proc. 58:35-39, 1983.

54. Nagasawa A, Kato K, Nishikawa K, Atsumi K, Arai K: Combined
    YAG Laser with CO$_2$ Laser Therapy Applied to Malignant Tumor.
    Abst. pres. at the 4th Congress of Int'l Society for Laser
    Surgery.   Tokyo, 11:38-41, 1981.

55. Oho K, Ohtani T, Amemiya R, Yamada R, Takei S, Taira O,
    Hayakawa K, Hayata Y: Laser Surgery in the Trachea and
    Bronchus via the Fiberoptic Bronchoscope.   Abst. from 4th
    Congress of Int'l Society for Laser Surgery, Tokyo. 14:16,
    1981.

56. Ohtani T, Takizawa N, Hayakawa K, Yamada R, Amemiya R, Oho K,
    Hayata Y: Role of Endoscopic Nd:YAG Laser Surgery in
    Staged Tracheoplasty.   Abst. Pres. at the 4th Congress of
    Int'l Society for Laser Surgery, Tokyo. 6:4, 1981.

57. Personne C, Colchen A, Toty L, Vourc'h G: Trachael Surgery
    Under Nd:YAG Laser.   Results of 521 Cases, 905 Sessions.
    Abst. Pres. at the 4th Congress of Int'l Society for Laser
    Surgery, Tokyo. 20:21, 1981.

58. Tamada J, Ito M, Teramatsu T: Clinical Study of Broncho-
    fiberscopic Nd:YAG Laser Surgery.   Abst. pres. at the 4th
    Congress of Int'l Society of Laser Surgery.   Tokyo.
    14:13-15,1981.

59. Toty L, Personne C, Colchen A, Vourc'h G: Trachael Surgery
    Under Nd:YAG Laser.   Necessity of Using a Modified Rigid
    Bronchoscope.   Abst. pres. at the 4th Congress of Int'l
    Society for Laser Surgery, Tokyo. 20:24, 1981.

60. Toty L, Personne C, Colchen A, Vourc'h G: Bronchoscopic Mgt.
    Of Trachael Lesions Using the Neodymium Yttrium Aluminum
    Garnet Laser.   Thorax 36:175-178, 1981.

61. Vouch'h G, Tannieres M, Toty L, Personne C: Anaestetic

Management of Trachael Surgery Using the Neodymium Yttrium Aluminum Garnet Laser. British Journal of Anaestesia. 52:993, 1980.

62. Yamada R, Amemiya R, Ohtani T, Taira O, Hayakawa K, Wada T, Ogawa I, Oho K, Hayata Y: Indications & Complications of Nd:YAG Laser Surgery via the Fiberoptic Bronchoscope in Cases Involving the Trachea & Major Bronchi. Abst. pres. the 4th Congress of Int'l Society for Laser Surgery. Tokyo, 6:21-24, 1981.

63. Saunders M, Young H, Becker D, Greenberg R, Newlon P, Corales R, Ham W, Povlishock J: The Use of the Laser in Neurological Surgery, Surgical Neurology, 14, July 1980.

64. Taki W, Takeuchi J, Yonekawa Y, Handa H: Advances in Laser Microsurgery in Neurosurgical Operations: With Special Reference to Nd:YAG Laser. Abst. pres. at the 4th Congress of Int'l Society of Laser Surgery, Tokyo. 18:15-17, 1981.

65. Goldrath M, Fuller T, Segal S: Laser Photovaporization of Endometrium for the Treatment of Menorrhagia. American Journal Obstet. Gynecology, 140(1):14-19, 1981.

66. Kozlov A, Moskalik K: Pulsed Laser Radiation Therapy of Skin Tumors. Cancer, 46(10):2172, 1980.

67. Lee T, Cho B, Park M: An Ultrastructural Study of the Cutaneous Pigmented and Vascular Lesions Treated by Nd:YAG Laser. Abst. pres. at the 4th Congress of Int'l Society of Laser Surgery, Tokyo. 24:17, 1981.

68. Noe J: Laser Use in Dermatology/Plastic Surgery. In Surgical Applications of Lasers by Dixon. Year Book Medical Publishers, Inc. 1983.

69. Dixon J: (1983) Surgical Application of Lasers. Year Book Medical Publishers, Inc. pg. 177.

70. Ibid. pg. 37.

71. Gulacsik C, Auth D, Silverstein F: Ophthalmic Hazards Associated With Laser Endoscopy. Applied Optics. 18:11, 1979.

72. Dixon J: (1983) Surgical Application of Lasers. Year Book Medical Publishers, Inc. pg. 37.

CHAPTER 26

DEVELOPMENT OF A LASER CENTER

Carolyn J. Mackety, R.N., B.S.
Director, Operating Room Services
Grant Hospital
111 South Grant Avenue
Columbus, Ohio 43215

DEVELOPMENT OF A LASER CENTER

AUTHOR: Carolyn J. Mackety, R.N., B.S.
Director, Operating Room Services
Grant Hospital
111 South Grant Avenue
Columbus, Ohio 43215
614/461-3096

To develop an effectively utilized program, various steps are necessary for implementation. Cost analysis in health care requires a careful
analysis and justification for each program as it is developed. With an
increasing number of lasers being installed in the operating room, the
Operating Room Director must be responsible for analyzing the program.
This analysis should include the cost effectiveness of the program, utilization review, space allocation, installation costs, procurement methods,
budget planning and control, development of job descriptions, a credentialing mechanism, safety requirements, monitoring external regulations,
evaluation of the program and marketing techniques.

A survey of the medical staff will result in commitment to use one of
the types of lasers being considered. Each physician should document this
intent and include a projected patient population, which is submitted to
the medical executive committee. Evaluation, input, and commitment to the
new laser program assists the overall corporate and long term strategic
planning. Based on the survey results, letters of intent, and program
commitment by administration, a medical staff committee should be appointed to monitor and evaluate the program on a regular basis.

The committee is comprised of physicians with considerable interest
and intent to use lasers in their practice. Included are representatives
from administration, nursing services, operating room services, and biomedical engineering. The purpose of the committee is laser selection;
policy and procedure development; credentialing mechanisms; education of
personnel to include physicians, nurses, and community; preventive maintenance of lasers, and finally, continous monitoring with evaluation of
the laser program.

When choosing the most appropriate laser for use in a multidiscipline
setting, the vendors present comprehensive information including an overview of state-of-the-art for that particular laser. General information
presented contains details of the warranty and service contracts that are
to be reviewed by the hospital attorney. The agreement includes an in
service for the hospital nursing units and probability of contractual
agreements for other services, such as a laser technician to be available
during interoperative procedures. When all the information and presenta-
tions have been obtained from the various laser companies, a decision is
made by the newly appointed laser committee together with the hospital
administration.

Several financial methods are available to obtain lasers. Outright
purchase is the most advantageous to the vendor and the hospital. With
recent emphasis on cost containment, other methods need to be considered.
Lease/purchase may be available either through the hospital's leasing
company with a lower interest rate, or through a leasing company at higher

© 1983 by Elsevier Science Publishing Co., Inc.
Neodymium-YAG Laser in Medicine and Surgery, Joffe, Muckerheide, and Goldman, editors

interest rates. Some laser companies will agree to place lasers in the hospital on a per use basis. This may initially appear cost effective, but when a cost analysis is completed, the hospital would probably not recoup its initial installation investment. However, this may be the only creative method of obtaining a laser at that time. A contractual agreement can have the user fee applied to the purchase price. Physicians have set up their own foundations for purchase of equipment. Agreements are contracted with the hospital for reimbursement based on laser usage. When developing this price structure, a percentage of the total charge is payable to the hospital. In a multi-use laser center, the ability to use creative financing may be important in making final decisions.

When lasers are purchased or procured, installation and accessory costs may not be included in the unit price. Installation and accessories can be costly and must be quoted in the purchase agreement. Carbon dioxide lasers require very little installation costs. It is however preferable that a separate circuit be installed so the electrical power is not interrupted during use. During most surgical procedures, several pieces of electrical equipment are often used. Plugging the laser into existing circuits may cause an overloading of the circuit. Furthermore, the Nd:YAG Laser requires a 208 volt, three phase power source. A power reducer may need to be installed in the laser. The Nd:YAG Laser also requires a continuous water source for cooling and drainage. The tuneable dye laser is immobile equipment and requires 440 volt, three phase electricity. Most operating rooms do not have this electrical power available and often requires installation to the local street power source. This laser is water cooled and the pump needs to be maintained at a constant pressure that may require a booster pump. A dye pump is necessary for the rhodamine dye which is mixed with methanol. A special trap in the sink must be installed for disposal of the waste dye. The tuneable dye laser is fixed equipment, and must be readily accessable to an operating room. Some renovation may be required. The newer lasers for ophthalmology, i.e. argon/krypton, and Nd:YAG are self contained units and can be used in a clinic or operating room setting.

When developing a budget for continued use of the laser, several items are taken into consideration. Carbon dioxide gas is used frequently and replaced regularly. A local medical gas vendor can be contracted to provide the special laser gas mixtures and deliver the cylinders on a monthly basis. Buying laser gas from the vendor is more expensive than using a local medical gas company. Projected use is analyzed and this cost is incorporated into the total laser charge. Other items that are patient charges are drapes for the laser, microscope, smoke evacuator, and quartz rods. Money should be budgeted for repair and replacement of instruments, fiberoptic equipment, and handpieces for the lasers. Service contracts are carefully considered and their cost is included in budget projections.

Accessories and instruments for laser use are important for continued and expanded use in each surgical discipline. It is suggested when using a CO_2 Laser that anodized instruments be used for safety. Several instrument companies have responded to this need at an increased cost. Maite instruments are readily available from most instrument companies at a reasonable cost and can be used with safety. The Nd:YAG is used with fiberoptics delivery systems and needs a complete complement of fiberscopes such as gastroscope, bronchoscope, and cystoscope. The endoscopes should be fitted with a white tip to prevent charing of the tip and need for replacement. The companies that are manufacturing the fiberscopes are currently beginning to respond to the need of the various instruments for laser surgery. The tuneable dye laser requires little instrumentation. However, as a laser used with fibers, the appropriate endoscope must be readily available. An important accessory is the laser fiber cutting and polishing kit. This saves cost in having to send the fibers out for continued repair. A person must be instructed in the methods of polishing and cutting of the fiber. The ophthalmology lasers require little instrumentation although a variety of lid retractors are available. The argon laser can be used with a handpiece for dermatology and special instruments may be required depending on the procedure.

The controller of each facility must take all costs into consideration for patient charges. The charge is not only based on cost, but patient use as initially projected in the utilization analysis completed during the feasibility study. The cost formula used is:

$$\frac{\text{Total Cost} \div \text{By Years of Amortization}}{\text{Projected Patient Use}} \times \% \text{ Increase} = \text{Patient Charge}$$

The percent of increase is based on direct and indirect costs. Direct cost includes gas, medical supplies, nursing and technician salaries. Indirect costs are utilities, renovation, and installation costs. Most patient charges for laser use have been approved by third party reimbursers. If the patient population changes, the laser charge can be adjusted to be cost effective.

For efficient operation of a multi-laser center, a team concept should be considered. A bio-laser technician undertakes the preventive maintenance, troubleshooting, and assists in setting each laser up for procedures, and is available as a laser safety technician. The bio-laser technician has graduated from a didactic and clinical program from a certified technical school. Although, not having a medical background, he has participated in a structured orientation program in the operating room.

The laser safety technician is dedicated for each laser procedure only to operate the laser in compliance with approved safety regulations. The safety technician sets up the laser, assists with draping, coupling laser to microscope, setting the power density with the surgeon, controls the power output and sets the machine on stand-by when not in use. When the procedure is complete, the safety technician shuts the laser down, cleans and stores lens, cleans fiberoptics, checks the laser, and carefully stores it. Also, working with the circulating nurse and scrub technician assures all equipment and supplies are readily available to meet the surgeons needs.

The clinical laser nurse's responsibility during the operative procedure would be similar to the laser safety technician. Her job includes the responsibility to do pre-operative visits on all laser patients. She also does post-operative evaluations and assesses each patient's satisfaction and progress.

The nurse's responsibility is to do patient assessment to meet the patient's and their family's needs during the surgical intervention. During the pre-operative visit, she takes the opportunity to reduce anxiety by discussing the operating room environment and pre- and post operative expectations. She explains to the patient the recovery room procedures and admitting process to the nursing unit. The family thus understands when the physician will be available to talk with them and especially where to wait until the patient returns to the nursing unit. She answers any questions they have about lasers and the application to the surgical procedure. Discussion concerning the actual surgical procedure is referred to the physician. A team conference is held with the operating room team to apprise them of special patient needs. The laser nurse sees the patients in the operating room prior to each procedure. Post-operative rounds are made by the nurse and her observations are documented on the multi-disciplinary notes. She also retains patient contact as needed and assists in discharge planning with the nursing unit.

For continued safe practice of lasers in surgery, each physician must have proper training in the use of each laser. Most didactic and clinical training available for physicians is approximately sixteen hours with accreditation for Category I CME's. Credentials should be filed with the medical staff secretary and available for verification, if needed. When the physician completes his training, the use of preceptors would be of assistance for the first few cases he performs. In-service training is important to understand how each laser is used and for continuing education, not only for physicians but also for nursing personnel. This type of training cannot take the place of hands-on animal laboratory training. Subsequently, "grandfathering" should not become a policy. All policies and procedures are developed and approved by the laser committee. Policies should include an approved credentialing mechanism. The method of documentation of laser use must include all pertinent information during the laser procedure. Data should include:

.Patient Name and I.D. Number
.Physician's Name
.Procedure Performed
.Power Density
.Information That Occurred During
The Procedure
.Time Elapsed

Informed consent, signed by each patient, should include that the procedure will be performed with the laser. Procedure cards are developed for each surgeon according to each surgical procedure where the laser is used.

Safety is of prime importance when using lasers. Firm safety policies should be established following the guidelines suggested for use of Class IV medical devices. These guidelines are published in ANSI standards and by the Bureau of Radiation Hazards. Although lasers do not have ionizing radiation, the hospital's radiation safety officer should be included in the development of safety rules. Each health care facility has a radiation safety officer who can assist in monitoring the laser safety. The bio-laser technician should become a member of the radiation safety committee. The proper eye protected glasses for each laser must be worn when the laser is activated. Glasses are different for each type of laser and with exception of the plastic glasses used during CO_2 procedures, the filtered glasses are very expensive. The endoscopes may also require filters for the eyepiece depending on which laser is used. Proper signs hung outside the operating room doors alerting personnel the laser is in use and proper safety precautions must be taken.

The Nd:YAG is considered an investigational device and is currently under the regulation of the F.D.A. The F.D.A. rules must be strictly followed and all protocols for use must have their approval. An investigator agreement must be signed in accordance with these regulations. Any changes in the established protocol must be approved by the principal investigators and the F.D.A. The reports that are generated gives the F.D.A. feedback as to the effectiveness of the device or treatment. Also, the F.D.A. compiles information and trends and keeps the investigator informed of progress with the device or treatment so the physician can update his knowledge and procedures. All investigational protocols are reviewed by the hospital's institutional review board for approval to be performed in that facility, and each protocol must have a method of evaluation stated. If the hospital does not have an investigational review board, the laser committee should review each protocol. When the protocols are reviewed by the committee, they are reviewed by the medical executive committee for approval. The approved protocol is then sent to the F.D.A.

The patient must sign an extensive informed consent with a certification statement signed by the principal investigating physician. The Federal Register has published the elements of informed consent that must be used by the physician. The nurses should understand the mechanism of investigational informed consent and make sure this consent is on the chart when the patient is sent to surgery.

Methods of evaluating a multi-laser clinical program are subjective. The accounting department can look at cost versus revenue generated. Medical records can trace the area of referral. The operating room can look at utilization, increased statistics and change in patient population. The nursing units can document patient care and satisfaction. The best method is to develop audit criteria and constantly evaluate the program as a whole. A computerized data base should help this evaluation mechanism.

Marketing a multi-laser center requires creative innovation, using cable television and newspaper articles. Short range marketing can include development of informational brochures with specific medical information fact sheets enclosed, sent to an identified physician population in a geographical referral base. Another good marketing technique is the development of laser seminars, workshops, and training courses. It is vitally important that the physician community know and understand what a multi-laser center is, but equally important is that the community know what the laser will be used for in medicine and surgery, and how it might ultimately be beneficial to them as an individual.

The development of a laser center requires time, education, and commitment. The medical staff must be committed to the development and use of the laser center. Administration must be visionary and be willing to take financial risks to provide new technology for improved patient care. There must be equipment and accessories and instrumentation to cover the scope of laser surgery for each surgical discipline.

The multi-laser center has the responsibility for education of physicians, nursing personnel, patients, and the community for the future practice of lasers in medicine and surgery.

CHAPTER 27

DOSIMETRY OF LASER ENERGY: SCIENCE VERSUS "WITCHCRAFT"

Principal Author:

Dan J. Castro, M.D.
Univ. of California, Los Angeles
Los Angeles, California

DOSIMETRY OF LASER ENERGY: SCIENCE VERSUS "WITCHCRAFT"

Dan J. Castro, M.D., and Patrick R. Abergel, M.D., and Malcolm A. Lesavoy, M.D.

INTRODUCTION

Historically, many ideas originate from coincidence. Intellectual curiosity and coincidence stimulated our introduction to the mysterious and fascinating world of laser. Sometime in September of 1979 while walking down the hallways of Harbor/UCLA Medical Center, we happened to witness Dr. Richard Dwyer performing a laser procedure. It first sounded like science fiction, but excited us to the point that we wanted to know more. After reading most of the published literature on lasers since 1961, and watching Dr. Dwyer working in his laser clinic, one of our first questions asked was, "How much energy is used by the laser?" His answer is still marked in our memory; "We don't have an accurate or reproducible method of dosimetry for laser energy". He continued, "But with experience, my eyes are trained to measure the amount of laser that should be delivered to tissues in order to obtain the desired results". Dr. Dwyer, as the other pioneers in this field, probably mastered the art of lasers so well, that they could "feel" what should be done. In the past four years, our group has been trying to find a solution to this fundamental but complicated problem. The first preliminary work has been published in the September, 1982 edition of the Annals of Plastic Surgery.[7] (This work was presented at the Fourth International Congress for Laser in Medicine and Surgery in Japan in 1981, and in the Second Annual Meeting of the American Society for Laser in Medicine and Surgery held in South Carolina in January, 1982). Our goals in the future is to develop the basic unit of dosimetry of laser absorbed energy, which we have termed the LAD (Laser Absortive Dose), analogous to the RAD in radiology.[5,6] In this book chapter, we will detail this scanning method of dosimetry which was developed in our laboratory at Harbor/UCLA Medical Center, with the help of the Department of Laser Physics at USC Medical Center. This method is simple, accurate (98%), reliable, and reproducible.[5,6,7] To date, researchers and clinicians have not used standardized methods. Using standardized laser dosimetry, data can be collected from various centers so that some sense can come out of "witchcraft".

PHYSICAL PRINCIPLES OF THE LASER

Laser is the acronym for Light Amplification by Stimulated Emission of Radiation. The laser is a high intensity light source which emits a nearly parallel electromagnetic beam of given wavelength generated in a suitable atomic or molecular system by means of a quantum optical process. The principles of induced or stimulated emission and their quantum optical foundations date back to Planck in 1908 and Einstein in 1917. We had to wait until 1954 and 1958 for Schawlow and Townes in the United States, and Prokhorov and Basov in the USSR to work out the physical principles of the MASER (Microwave Amplification by Stimulated Emission of Radiation),[2,10,25] and thereby pave the way for its application to the shorter light wave. After extensive preliminary theoretical work, Maiman (in 1960)[19,20] in the United States became the first to operate a solid laser using a chromium ruby crystal. The first gas laser, a Helium-neon Laser, was developed by Javan, Bennet, and Herriott (1961)[1,2,11,14] the crystal Neodymium-YAG Laser, by Jonson and Nassau 1961,[8,18,26] and finally the CO_2 gas laser by Patel in 1964.[23]

© 1983 by Elsevier Science Publishing Co., Inc.

Neodymium-YAG Laser in Medicine and Surgery, Joffe, Muckerheide, and Goldman, editors

GENERATION OF LASER BEAMS

The basic concept of the quantum theory[13,31] states that atomic or molecular systems can be in two various energy states, the first of which is their normal or basal energy state known as the ground state. The second known as the "excited state" is attained at various higher energy levels, by the addition of thermal, electrical, chemical, or radiation energy stimulation. An atomic or molecular system "excited" in this way reverts to its own energy level either by radiation after some time in this state (spontaneous emission), or by interaction with external incident radiation whose wavelength corresponds to the energy absorbed (stimulated emission) emitting a beam of photons. In such an atomic or molecular system, the number of excited states is sufficiently large for an incident wavelength to produce more induced emission with absorption process (inversion state). The energy released can be amplified by a beam (amplification by stimulated emission). In the laser medium, i.e., gas, solid, or liquid state in which the excited state reverts to the ground or basal state, (by emitting photons) a sufficient number of atomic or molecular systems can be excited by the uptake of an energy pump (electrical, thermal or chemical) to obtain the state of inversion.[17] The beam thus produced, undergoes multiple reflections along the axis between the two parallel mirrors forming a resonator, and is amplified with each passage through the medium. One part of the laser beam so produced escapes through a partially transparent resonator. In this way, an infinite number of laser systems can be produced. We can distinguish among the four major categories of lasers according to the state of aggregation of the laser material or according to the way in which the energy required for inversion is obtained. There are solid state lasers, liquid lasers, gas lasers, and free electron lasers.

The wavelengths of laser beams of the individual systems cover the light spectrum from the near ultraviolet region to the far infrared region.[9]

The Neodymium-YAG Laser is a solid state laser, made from a crystal yttrium aluminum garnet crystal ($Y_3AL_5O_2$) with incorporated (ion doped) $Nd3+$ of certain concentration. These ions are excited by the absorption of light energy. It is accomplished by focusing the light from a discharge lamp, (Krypton lamps of 1000 watts each) on to the rod-like crystal by a suitable system of electrical cylindrical mirrors (optical pumps). The resonator may be arranged directly on the end surfaces of the cylindrical crystal or positioned away from them.

For the argon laser, the argon gas is placed within a tube that contains reflective mirrors at the ends of this tube. A high electrical voltage is then passed through this tube so that electrons in the outer orbits of the argon laser are raised to high energy levels for a short period of time.

When these electrons revert back down to their normal ground energy state, they each emit a photon of light of a specific wavelength or color. These photons are then reflected back and forth between the mirrors at the ends of the "argon tube", and in so doing, they strike and collide with other excited argon atoms. This causes a build-up of photons of the same wavelength. Subsequently, this group of photons are allowed to exit the tube, and this results in a monochromatic, in-phase, energy laser (light). Subsequently, this laser energy (light) can be directed with various focusing lenses in a fiber optic pathway to a hand piece which can then be directed at various targets.

Depending on the operative mode of the laser system, the energy may first, be stored briefly, and the beam then emitted in the form of discrete pulses (pulse or super pulse laser), or there may be a continuous ouput of energy (continuous wave characteristics of Neodymium-YAG Laser).

As a result of the processes described above, the laser irradiation produced has three essential properties: 1) Monochromaticity (pure color); 2) Parallel light beams; 3) Coherence.

It is known, though, that when any laser beam is transmitted through a fiber optic, it looses its coherent property.[3,4,15,16,29,30] It means that one of the most important single properties of the laser is in its monochromaticity, which results in different extinction factors in tissues, according to each laser's wavelength. The extinction factor (Gama Γ) or the total change in intensity of the laser tissues, is equal to the sum of the absorption (α) and scattering (β) of the beam, and follows the Lambert Beer's Law. (Table I)

$$I = Ioe^{-\Gamma L}$$

This law expresses the fact that the beam intensity (power density) referred to the initial intensity Io of the incident beam, decreases exponentially with the depth L in the tissue.

The absorption power (α) describes the decrease in the radiation power per unit of path length.

The term scattering (β) refers to the angular divergence undergone by a beam of light onpassing through its target.

IN CONCLUSION:

Different Wavelengths = Different Specific Extinction Factors = Different Biological Changes in Tissue.

The above facts are true for the three main lasers used today. Previous experiments done before[12] have shown that in water and gastric mucosa the extinction coefficient, vascular coagulation and depth of penetration, for the CO_2, Argon and Neodymium-YAG Lasers are distinctly different (Table I).

From Table I, it is easy to understand why the CO_2 Laser is the "best" scalpel, but it has limited vascular coagulation capacities. The Neodymium-YAG Laser, though, because of its absorption capacities and high scattering factors, is the "best" coagulator and has a unique capacity of deep tissue penetration. These specific properties of the Neodymium-YAG Laser gives hope for possibilities of the broad spectrum of biological changes in human tissues.[5,6]

"FACTS"? FROM THE PAST MEDICAL LITERATURE

Many published data in the past medical literature has been based on incorrect assumptions. For example, it is commonly written: 1)"The distribution of laser energy in tissue is uniform, and has a Guaussian shape distribution". The calculated surface of a circular-shaped light spot is equal to πr^2, (r=radius of the circle). So by measuring the diameter of the light spot on the target, the surface could be easily calculated, the power density and the energy density could then be derived. Unfortunately, this fact is only true for single mode lasers (Helium-neon for example), and not for most of the lasers used in medicine, (CO_2, Argon, Neodymium-YAG) which are all multimode lasers. It is an accepted fact in laser physics[21,22,24,27,28] that multimode laser and optical fibers create a non-uniform and complicated beam spatial distribution. This means that the beam profile is complex and is not the assumed Guaussian distribution.[7] That's why the circle-shaped surface of the laser spot is not equal to πr^2, but in fact has to be integrated ($S = \int_0^r 2\pi r \, Fc(r)dr$).

2) <u>Way of measurement of laser spot diameter on the target</u>. The
Neodymium-YAG Crystal Laser and CO_2 Gas Laser have wavelengths respectively
of 10,600Å, and 106,000Å, which are near and in the mid infrared spectrum.
These two laser beams are <u>invisible,</u> and most manipulators would then either
calculate the diameter of the pilot light on the target (Helium-neon laser,
wavelength of 6324Å, which has a red color in the visible spectrum) and/or
the diameter of a burn-treated spot.

This type of measurement is inaccurate and non-reproducible. Because
of the difference in wavelengths between the pilot light (Helium-neon) and
the laser beams (Neodymium-YAG or CO_2), the spatial distribution, the di-
fraction factors, the beam divergence, the focal points from the fiber outlet to the target are <u>different</u>. That means that the spot diameter on the
target at any distance from the fiber optic or hand piece <u>must</u> be different
from the pilot light.

Another source of inaccuracies is that the diameter of the burned spot
by laser light energy source varies with multiple factors; i.e., type of
laser used, time of exposure and tissue or material exposed: This is so
because of the variance of the extinction factors with the differing modes
of lasers (Beer's Law). (Table I)

INSTRUMENTATION

1) Laser

The laser used is a standard continuous wave (CW) Neodymium-YAG (Neo-
dymium:Yttrium Aluminum Garnet) Crystal Laser$^{(Fig.I)}$ from MBB-AT Company,
with a wavelength of 10,600Å (invisible, near infrared), and a maximal power
output of 60 watts. The pilot light is a Helium-neon gas (2mV, with a wavelength of 6324Å, visible, red color).

2) Beam Scanner

It is a simple device which can be built by any user.$^{(Fig. II)}$ The
translation stage $^{(Fig. II,4)}$ is composed of two metal plates distant from
each other by an aperture of 57μ .$^{(Fig.II,5)}$ $^{(Fig.III,5)}$ It has been determined through extensive calculations that a slit with a width not exceeding
½ the radius of the laser beam may be used as the aperture without introducing important errors.[7,28] This translation stage is driven by a micrometer Model 263 (Starret Co., Massachusetts, USA)$^{(Fig. II,3)}$ which is connected to a standard motor (110 volts) which rotates the micrometer constantly at 12 rotations per minute.$^{(Fig. II,1)}$

At each rotation of the micrometer, the translation stage is driven by
0.025 inches or 0.0634 centimeters.

3) Power Meter

A coherent thermopile 210$^{(Fig. IV)}$ is used to measure the average power
of the laser beam. This meter is sensitive enough to be utilized as the detector of the beam scanner. The instrument consists of a compact direct absorption head (easily detached).$^{(Fig. IV,4)}$ An adjustable stand, and a
battery operated control indicator unit is available.$^{(Fig. IV,1)}$ The model
210 features broadband sensitivity (UV to infrared), with ±5% accuracy. The
response meter$^{(Fig. IV,2)}$ ranges of 03,1.0,3.0., and 10.0 watts are selected
with a front panel rotary switch.$^{(Fig.IV,3)}$ A simple standard power multiplier (high speed rotating blade, with a multiplying factor of 9.52 is used,
when the power output is greater than 10 watts.

4)   Chart Recorder

A standard chart recorder, Model 156 (Fig. V,1) from Cole Parmer Instrument Co., is used in our laboratory. This chart recorder (110 volts) is controlled by an ON and OFF switch. (Fig. V,2) Switch speed (Fig. V,3) controls the speed of the millimeter recording paper (Fig. V,5) (variable from 2-20 centimeters/minute or centimeters/hour). Another switch "input" (Fig. V,4) controls the sensitivity of recording, variable from one millivolt to 10 volts.

METHOD

The beam scan is a popular technique in laser physics used to measure a spatial profile of the laser beam [7,24,27] The experimental apparatus is outlined in Fig. VI. The mounted apparatus is shown in Fig. VII. The laser beam (hand piece or fiber optics) is fixed at a measured distance from the translation stage. (Fig. VII,3) This distance is decided by the manipulator and varies depending upon the desired spot surface, and energy density. The laser ouput passes through the aperture or slit (Fig. II,5) which is mounted on the translation stage (Fig. VIII,2) The micrometer drive on the translation stage moves the aperture in a direction which is perpendicular to the direction of the beam propagation. The light transmitted through this aperture (slit) is sensed by a detector also mounted on the translation stage (Fig. VII,5) which is connected to a chart recorder (Fig. VII,9) which records the beam profile. The laser beam can be compared to an "orange", which is "sliced" by the beam scanner, (Fig. II) the power sensor (Fig. IV,4) detects each "orange slice" and records it on the chart recorder which "reconstructs" the orange shape.

The measured beam profile, (Fig. VIII) registered by the chart recorder, may be used to determine the peak intensity of the incident laser light.

HOW TO RECORD THE BEAM

Step I

Once the Neodimium-YAG Laser is turned on (Fig. I,2) the apparatus is mounted as shown in picture; (Fig. VII) measure and then fix the hand piece or fiber optic at the desired distance from the translation stage. (Fig.VII,3) This will be defined as the distance of hand piece parameter (DHP).
- Keep the hand piece or fiber optic at 90° from the translation stage.

  - Be sure that the pilot light (Helium-neon) is distant laterally at least 2 cm. from the slit (aperture) on the translation stage. (Fig. VII,4)

Step II

1) Turn the rotary switch on the power meter (Fig. IV, 3) (Fig. VII, 7) to one of the positions on the dial (variable from 0.3 to 10.0 watts).

2) Turn the dial input on the chart recorder (Fig. V, 4)(Fig. VII, 9) to one of the positions (variable from 0.1 to 100 millivolts).

3) Turn the switch speed of paper (Fig. V, 3) (Fig. VII, 9) on the chart recorder to one of the desired speeds (variable from 2 to 20 cm. per minute).

By adjusting these switches on the power meter and on the chart recorder, we are able to find at any desired distance of hand piece or distance of the fiber optics from the translation stage the most sensitive recording capacity which allows one to record the "highest" and "widest" beam shape. Therefore, this will facilitate the statistical analysis of the recorded beam.

4) Turn the chart recorder switch$^{(Fig. \ V,2)}$ to the ON position. Calibrate the recording pen on the chart recorder to the zero line$^{(Fig.V,5)}$ (a straight line should be recorded on the 1cm. line.)

5) Turn the beam scanner switch$^{(Fig. \ VII, \ 1)}$ to the ON position and the micrometer on the beam scanner$^{(Fig. \ II, \ 3)}$ will start driving the translation stage in a direction which is perpendicular to the laser propagation.

Step III

- Push on the foot pedal of the Neodymium-YAG Laser.$^{(Fig. \ I,5)}$
- Recalibrate the recording pen on the chart recorder to the zero line.$^{(Fig.V,5)}$ As mentioned in Step I, the Neodymium-YAG Laser spot was kept at a lateral distance from the slit on the translation stage,$^{(Fig.VII,4)}$ so that the recording of the entire spot of the laser beam is accomplished. At this step the Neodymium-YAG Laser beam is ON, and the translation stage is moving in a direction which is perpendicular to the laser beam propagation stage, and the chart recorder should first record a straight line. Once the edges of the Neodymium-YAG Laser beam start to pass through the aperture (slit) it will be sensed by the power sensor,$^{(Fig.VII,5)}$ and then recorded on the chart recorder paper.$^{(Fig.VII,9)}$ First, by an ascending loop up to a maximum (which corresponds to a center of the laser beam spot), and then to a descending loop, until again a straight line will be recorded on the chart recorder paper,$^{(Fig.VIII)}$ meaning that the entire Neodymium-YAG Laser spot was scanned. This step should be repeated, in order to obtain at least 5 recorded beams at any fixed distance of hand piece from the translation stage. This will allow a valid statistical analysis of the desired calculated parameters.

Step IV

Turn off the Neodymium-YAG Laser, the beam scanner, the power meter, and the chart recorder.

HOW TO ANALYZE A BEAM

The measured beam profile, as registered by the chart recorder,$^{(Fig.VIII)}$ may be used to determined the peak intensity of the laser light. Numerical integration has been used to analyze the measured profile to obtain the peak intensity.[7] The formula used in the analysis is:

$$Po = Io \int_0^\infty 2\pi r Fc(r) dr$$

Where Po is the total power in watts, Fc(r) is the spatial distribution taken from the chart recorder normalized to unity, and Io is the peak intensity axis of the beam in watts/^{2}cm.

A. Calculation of the surface (S) of the laser beam spot.

The formula used in the analysis is:

$$S= \int_0^{\infty} 2\pi rFc(r)dr$$

Step 1.   Measure the maximum distance ab in centimeters between the base of the ascending and descending loop of the registered curve, and draw a straight line. (Fig.VIII) Divide the distance in half (point c, Fig. VIII) and draw a perpendicular line (dc, Fig. VIII), which should divide the peak of the registered beam in the center. Each half of the beam can be used in the surface calculation.

Step 2.   Divide the distance ac (Fig. VIII), into an <u>even</u> number of units. The distance between each unit is constant and is defined as r (Fig. VIII). In this example the r is equal to o.5 cm., and the number of units chosen is 12 (even number). (Chosen arbitrarily by the manipulator). Draw a perpendicular line to each corresponding r (Fig. VIII).

Step 3.   Measure the height dc, defined as f(r), Fig. VIII). This is equal to the height in centimeters.

Step 4.   To each r (Fig. VIII) (Fig. IX,5) measure the corresponding f(r) (Fig. VIII) (Fig. IX,6) and calculate the corespondent Fc(r) (Fig. IX,7) and y (Fig.IX,8) using the mathematical formula as shown above. (Fig. IX)

Step 5.   Simpson's rule mathematical formula (Fig. IX, 9) was used to evaluate the above data, to obtain the surface spot(S) (Fig. IX,10) The value of the surface is expressed in cm^2

B.   Calculation of the spot diameter of the laser beam.

1.   FWHM (Full Width Half Maximum)
Derived from Beer's Law, (Table I) equal to the spot diamter at 50% of the peak intensity of the laser beam. At 50% of value of f(r) (Fig.VIII,m) measure the number of units on the graph paper between k1 and multiply this value by the correcting factor (Fig.VIII) (Fig. IX,11) This value is expressed in centimeters.

2.   1/e
Derived also from Beer's Law (Table I), is equal to the spot diameter at 37% of the peak intensity of the laser beam (Beer's Law, when L=1/Υ). Calculate 37% of the values of f(r) (Fig.VIII,j) Measure at this point the number of units on the graph paper between points ih. Multiply this value by the correcting factor (Fig. VIII) (Fig. IX,12) This value is expressed in centimeters.

3. $1/e^2$
This is equal to the spot diameter at 14% of the peak intensity of the laser beam. (Beer's Law) When L=2/Υ) (Table I) Calculate 14% of the value of f(r) (Fig. VIII,g) Measure the number of units on the graph paper between points ef. Multiply this value by the correcting factor. (Fig. VIII) (Fig. IX, 13) This value is expressed in centimeters.

C.   Measurements of power and time of exposure.
1.   The power output of the laser is variable. It is measured using the power meter Model 210 (Fig. IV) and power multiplier. This value is expressed in watts.

2. The time of exposure is controlled with a time shutter $^{(Fig. IV)}$ and This value is expressed in seconds.

D. Calculation of the intensity (or Irradiance, or power density). By definition the intensity is equal to the laser power output divided by the surface of the laser spot or:

$$Io= \frac{Po}{\int_{o}^{\infty} 2\pi rFc(r)dr}$$

This value is expressed in watts/cm^2

E. Calculation of the energy density or energy fluence. The energy density is equal to the product of the intensity (I) and time of exposure.

$$\text{Energy density} = \frac{\text{Laser Power Output(watts)} \cdot \text{Time of Exposure (seconds)}}{\text{Surface(cm}^2)}$$

This value is expressed in Joules/cm^2

REQUIRED PARAMETERS IN THE CHAPTER "MATERIAL AND METHODS".

In too many of the published articles on lasers in medicine and surgery, the chapter "Material and Methods" is lacking indispensable data. In more than 90% of past articles, one has an impossible effort to reproduce similar findings. We find this fact regretable, since most of the published results are very exciting for the future uses of lasers in clinical medicine and surgery.

In order to standardize laser work among researchers and clinicians around the world, this chapter should be detailed.

Needed published data are:

1. Type of laser (company, wavelength).
2. Mode of laser (CW, Pulse, Super pulse).
3. Maximal power output of the laser (watts).
4. Type of hand piece or fiber optic used.
5. Focal point (millimeter) of the fiber optic or hand piece used.
6. Distance of the hand piece or fiber optic from the treated target (centimeter). Kept constant or variable?
7. Measured power at time of use of the laser, and type of power meter used.
8. Time of exposure of each single laser pulse.
9. Angle of incidence of the fiber optic or hand piece.
10. Calculated spot diameter at FWHM, 1/e, 1/e^2, in centimeter.
11. Calculated intensity (I) in watts/cm^2.
12. Calculated energy density, Joules/cm^2.
13. Anatomical treated area, and type of treated lesion.
14. Total surface in cm^2 of laser treated area.
15. Total number of laser treated spots.
16. Distance in mm. between each laser treated spots.
17. Total number, and time intervals between each laser treatment.
18. Length of follow up.

"LAD"

The rapid increase of clinical and research uses of lasers around the world, has made the introduction of the "LAD" indispensable. In the future, we feel it will be the basic unit of absorption of laser energy in tissues.[5,6] The "LAD" (Laser Absorptive Dose) is parallel to the RAD in radiology, and will be equal to 100 erg/cm^3. The mathematical formula for the LAD is also derived from Beer's Law.

$$1 \text{ LAD} = \frac{PoXto(1-e^{-\Upsilon L})}{L \int_{o}^{\infty} 2\pi rFc(r)dr}$$

In this chapter, we have described a simple, accurate, and reproducible method of dosimetry of laser energy per surface area. The LAD will measure the amount of laser energy per volume or gram absorbed in specific tissue. Our laboratory is currently developing a simple and reproducible technique of measurement of the extinction factor (Υ) and the depth of penetration (L) of laser energy in different specific tissues, and therefore the LAD will become a reality.

CONCLUSION:

By using this simple and accurate method of measurement of spot diameter, intensity and energy densities, we are able to reproduce similar histological damage to any tissue by using the different energy sources of the Neodymium-YAG Laser, as well as the Argon or CO_2 Lasers.[7] Previously, clinicians and technicians just turned the machine to low, medium, or high and delivered virtually unknown quantities of energy to a particular amount of tissue. No scientific study can be made to determine the biological effects of the medical laser energy source without first documenting the amount of energy delivered to a particular tissue. The method of dosimetry described in this chapter is the first small step which can allow standardization of work with any laser energy source, until the birth of the "LAD".

$$\boxed{I = I_0\, e^{-\gamma L}} \qquad \boxed{\gamma = \alpha + \beta}$$

$\alpha\,[cm^{-1}] =$ ABSORPTION COEFFICIENT

$\frac{1}{\alpha}\,[cm] =$ PENETRATION DEPTH

LASER	$\frac{1}{\alpha}[cm^{-1}]$	VASCULAR COAGULATION Φ OF VESSEL	COEFFICIENT $= \dfrac{\text{ABSORPTION }(\alpha)}{\text{SCATTERING }(\beta)}$	TISSUE
Nd-YAG-LASER $\lambda = 1.06\,\mu m$	$\frac{1}{12}$ cm = 0.8 mm	> 1.5 mm	$\frac{\alpha}{\beta} \ll 1$	LIVER STOMACH SKIN
ARGON-LASER $\lambda = 0.5\,\mu m$	$\frac{1}{50}$ cm = 0.2 mm	$\approx$ 0.8 mm	$\frac{\alpha}{\beta} = 1$	
CO_2-LASER $\lambda = 10\,\mu m$	$\frac{1}{200}$ cm = 0.05 mm	$\approx$ 0.5 mm	$\frac{\alpha}{\beta} \gg 1$	

Table 1. Depth of penetration, vascular coagulation, absorption over scattering coefficient for the Nd:YAG, Argon and CO_2 Lasers.

256

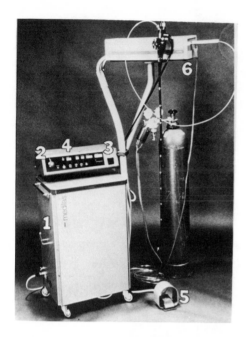

Fig. 1. Nd:YAG (Neodymium:Yttrium Aluminum Garnet)
1. Power Supply
2. Power ON-OFF Keylock switch
3. Power Meter
4. Time shutter
5. Foot pedal
6. Laser unit

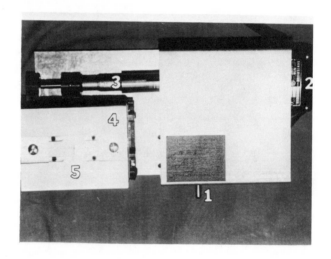

Fig. 2. BEAM SCANNER
1. ON and OFF switch
2. Standard Motor (11 volts)
3. Micrometer Model 263
4. Translation stage
5. Slit or aperture

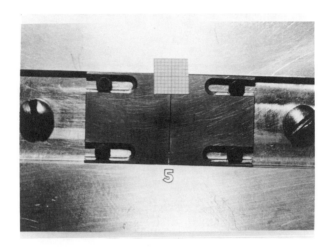

Fig. 3. Top view of translation
stage
5 - slit or aperture of 57μ

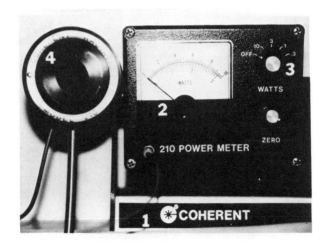

Fig. 4. Coherent thermopile 210
1. Battery operated indicator
2. Response meter
3. Rotary switch
4. Absorption head, or power
   sensor used also as detector
   of the Beam Scanner.

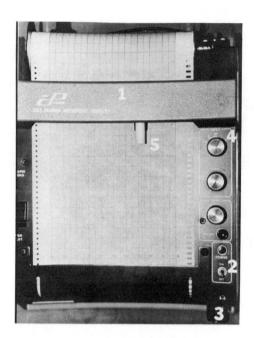

Fig. 5. - Chart recorder Model 156
1. Chart recorder, 110V, Cole
   Parmer Instrument Co.
2. ON and OFF switch
3. Switch speed recording paper
4. Switch, INPUT, sensitivity
   of recording.

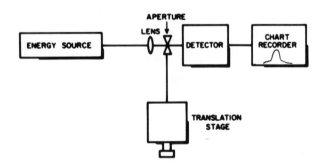

Fig. 6. Experimental Apparatus

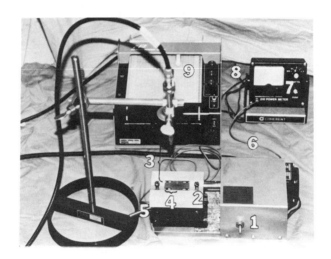

Fig. 7. - Mounted experimental apparatus

1. ON and OFF switch on Beam Scanner
2. Translation stage
3. Distance Hand Piece (DHP)
4. Lateral initial distance from slit (aperture),
   at least 2 cm.
5. "Hand" of Power Sensor (kept under slit)
6. Connection between Power Sensor to Power Meter
7. Power Meter Model 210
8. Connection between Power Meter to Chart Recorder
9. Chart Recorder Model 156

260

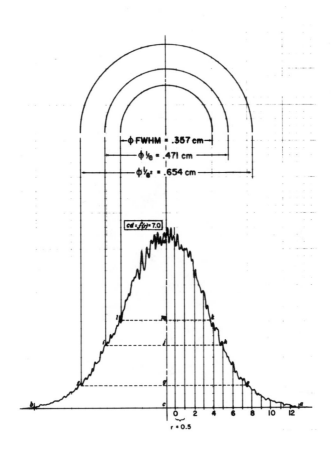

Fig. 8.   Measured Beam Profile

$r=o$ (5)	$f(r)=7.0$ (6)	14 (7) $F(r) \dfrac{f(n)\ (r)}{f(r)} \text{XCF}^{(1)}$	$y=2\pi r f(r)dr$ (8)
$r_o=.5$	$f_o\ (r)=6.7$	$F_o\ (r)=.073$	$y_o=.229$
$r_1=1.5$	$f_1\ (r)=6.4$	$F_1\ (r)=.069$	$y_1=.433$
$r_2=2.0$	$f_2\ (r)=5.4$	$F_2\ (r)=.059$	$y_2=.556$
$r_3=2.5$	$f_3\ (r)=4.65$	$F_3\ (r)=.050$	$y_3=.628$
$r_4=3.0$	$f_4\ (r)=3.3$	$F_4\ (r)=.036$	$y_4=.565$
$r_5=3.5$	$f_5\ (r)=2.55$	$F_5\ (r)=.028$	$y_5=.528$
$r_6=4.0$	$f_6\ (r)=1.8$	$F_6\ (r)=.020$	$y_6=.440$
$r_7=4.5$	$f_7\ (r)=1.15$	$F_7\ (r)=.012$	$y_7=.301$
$r_8=5.0$	$f_8\ (r)=.7$	$F_8\ (r)=.088$	$y_8=.226$
$r_9=5.5.$	$f_9\ (r)=.5$	$F_9\ (r)=.005$	$y_9=.157$
$r_{10}=6.0$	$f_{10}(r)=.3$	$F_{10}(r)=.003$	$y_{10}=.104$
$r_{11}=6.0$	$f_{11}(r)=.2$	$F_{11}(r)=.002$	$y_{11}=.075$
$r_{12}=6.5$	$f_{12}(r)=.1$	$F_{12}(r)=.001$	$y_{12}=.041$

$$S=1/3h^{(2)} \left[y_o+2y_2+4y_3+\ldots\ldots+4y_{(n-1)}+y_{(n=even)} \right] \quad (9)$$

$$S=1/3 \left[o.5(.076)\right]\left[\begin{array}{l} .229+4(.433)+2(.556)+4(.628)+2(.565)+4(.528)+2(.440) \\ +4(.301)+2(226)+4(.157)+2(.104)+4(.073)+.041 \end{array} \right] \quad (10)$$

$$S=.159 \text{cm}^2$$

$\emptyset^{(4)}_{\text{FWHM}}=.357$ cm. (11)

$\emptyset^{(4)}_{1/e}=.471$ cm. (12)

$\emptyset^{(4)}_{1/e^2}=.654$ cm. (13)

1. CF= Correcting Factor – Correcting Factor (CF): Correct the values of r to real measured values in centimeters. The correcting factor is equal to the product of the number of RPM of the micrometer (Constant=12 RPM) by the distance of the translation stage driven by each rotation of the micrometer (Constant=0.0635cm.) This value divided by the speed of the recording paper on the chart recorder (variable from 2 to 20 cm/minute).

2. h=rxCF
9. Simpson's Rule Mathematical Formula
4. Diameter ($\emptyset$)=Number of Units X CF

Fig. 9.

262

REFERENCES

1. Bennett, W.R., Jr.: "Inversion Mechanisms in Gas Lasers", Appl., Opt., Suppl. 2 Chem. Laser, 3-33, 1965.

2. Bennett, W.R., Jr.: "Gaseous Optical Masers," Applied Opt., Suppl. Opt. Masers, 24-64, 1962.

3. Boyd, G.D., and Gordon, J.P.: "Confocal Multimode Resonator for Millimeter through Opitcal Wavelength Masers," Bell Syst. Tech. J. 40, 489-508, March, 1961.

4. Boyd, G.D., and Kogelnik, H.:"Generalized Confocal Resonator Theory," Bell Syst. Tech, J. 41, 1347-1369, July, 1962.

5. Castro, D.J., Abergel, R.P., Johnston, K.J., Adomian, G.E., Dwyer, R.M., Uitto, J., Lesavoy, M.A.: Wound Healing: Biological Effects of Nd:YAG Laser on Collagen Metabolism in Pig Skin in Comparison to Thermal Burn. Ann. Plastic Surgery (in press).

6. Castro, D.J., Abergel, R.P., Meeker, C., Dwyer, R.M., Lesavoy, M.A., Uitto, J.: Effect of the Nd:YAG Laser on DNA Synthesis and Collagen Production in Human Skin Fibroblast Cultures. Ann. Plastic Surgery (in press).

7. Castro, D.J., Benvenuti, D., Dwyer, R., Lesavoy, M.A.: A New Method of Dosimetry. Study of Comparative Laser-Induced Tissue Damage. Ann. Plastic Surgery 9: 221-226, 1982.

8. Danielmey, H.G.: "Progress in YAG Lasers," in Lasers, Vol. 4 ed. A.K. Levine and A.J. DeMaria (New York: Marcel Dekker, Inc. 1976), P. 8.

9. Eden, J.G., Burnjam, R., Champagne, L.F., Donohue, T., DJeu, N.: Visible and UV Lasers: Problems and Promises," IEEE Spectrum, 50-59, April, 1979.

10. Fox, A.G., Li, T.: "Resonant Modes in a Maser Interferometer," Bell Syst. Techn. J. 40, 453-488, March, 1961.

11. Herriott, D.R.: "Applications of Laser Light", Sci. Am. 219, 141-156, 1968.

12. Hofstetter, A., and Frank, F.: The Nd:YAG Laser in Urology. Roche, Basle, Switzerland, 1-72, 1980.

13. Holonyak, N.Jr., Kolbas, R., Dupris, R.D., Dapkus, P.D.: "Quantum Well Heterostructrue Lasers,", IEEEJ. of Wunat. Electr. Qe-16, 170-180, 1980.

14. Javan, A., Bennett, W.R, Jr., and Herriott, D,R.: "Population Inversion and Continuous Optical Maser Oscillation in Gas Discharge Containing a He-Ne Mistures," Phys. Rev. 6, 106, 1961.

15. Kogelnik, H.: "Imaging of Optical Modes-Resonators with Internal Lenses," Bell Syst. Techn. J. 44, 455-494, March, 161.

16. Kogelnik, H., and Li, T.: "Laser Beams and Resonators", Appl. Opt. 5, 1550-1556, Oct. 1966.

17. Koechner, W., DeBenedictis, L.C., Matovich, E., and Meyer, G.E.:
    "Characteristics and Performance of High Power CW Krypton Arc
    Lamps for Nd:YAG Laser Pumping,: IEEE J. Quant. Electron. Q-E, 8,
    310, 1972.

18. Kushida, T., Marcos, H.M., and Geusic, J.E.: "Laser Transition
    Cross-section and Fluorescence Branching Ratio for Nd^{3+} in Yttrium
    Aluminum Garnet," Phys. Ed. 167, 1289, 1969.

19. Maiman, T.: "Stimulated Optical Emission in Fluroscent Solids I.
    Theoretical Consideration", Phys. Rev. 123, 1145-1150, Aug. 15,
    1961.

20. Mainman, T., Hoskins, R.H., D'Haenens,I.J., Asawa, C.K., and
    Evtuhov, V.: "Stimulated Optical Emission in Fluorescent Solids.
    II Spectroscopy and Stimulated Emission in Ruby," Phys. Rev. 123,
    1151-1157, Aug. 15,1967.

21. Maitland A., and Dunn, M.H.: Laser Physics (Amsterdam: North-
    Holland Publishing Compnay, 1972)

22. Marcuse, D.: Light Transmission Optics (Princeton, N.J.: D. Van
    Nostrand Company, 1972).

23. Patel,C.K.N.: "High Power Carbon Dioxide Lasers," Sci. Am. 219,
    22-23, 1968.

24. Selby, S.M. (ed.): Stand Mathematical Tables. Cleveland,
    Chemical Rubber Company, 1969, P. 14.

25. Siegman, A.E.: An Introduction to Lasers and Masers (New York:
    McGraw-Hill Book Company, 1971).

26. Streetman, B.G.: Solid State Electronic Devices, 2nd Ed.
    (Englewood Cliffs, N.J.: Prentice-Hall, Inc., 1980). Chap. 10.

27. Suzaki, Y. Tachibana, A.: Applied Optics L4:2809, 1975.

28. Van Stryland, E.W., Bass, M., Soileau, M.H., et al.: Laser
    Induced Damages in Optical Material, 1977. In Glass AJ,
    Guenther (eds.), National Bureau of Standardization Special
    Publication 509. Washington, DC, US Government Printing
    Offices, 1978, P. 118.

29. Verdeyen, J.T.: Laser Electronics, Prentice-Hall Inc.
    Englewood Cliffs, New Jersey, 1968.

30. Yariv, A.: Introduction to Optical electronics, 2nd ed.
    (New York: Holt, Rinehart and Winston, 1971), Chap. 7.

31. Yariv, A.: Quantum electronics 2nd ed. (New York, John Wiley
    and Sons, Inc., 1975), Chap. 10.

CHAPTER 28

EFFECTS OF LASER SOURCES ON THE ELASTIC RESISTANCE

OF THE VESSEL WALLS

Principal Author:

Victor Aldo Fasano
Unstitute of Neurosurgery
University of Turin
Torino, Italy

EFFECTS OF LASER SOURCES ON THE ELASTIC RESISTANCE OF THE VESSEL WALLS

Victor Aldo Fasano, Roberto Maria Ponzio and Franco Benech
Institute of Neurosurgery, University of Turin, via Cherasco
15, 10126 Torino, Italia.

INTRODUCTION

The function of the elastic elements of the vessel wall is to produce a tension suitable to resist the distention strength made by blood pressure. By producing a modification in the morphologic and structural configuration of such elastic elements it is possible to obtain changes in the elastic resistance of the wall. The purpose of this investigation is the recording of the elastic behavior of blood vessels before and after laser irradiation.

MATERIALS AND METHODS

Forty rabbits weighing 2 to 3 kg were anesthetized with ethylurethan (1 g/Kg IV) or nembutal (35 mg/Kg IV). The femoral vein was catheterized and trachea cannulated. Both carotid arteries were isolated. Two series of experiments have been performed in both acute and chronic stage. In the first one the artery was placed between a perfusing system with saline solution (B. Braun Melsungen mod. Perfusor) and a merqury nanometer; an intraluminal pressure of 30 mm Hg was produced. The vessel diameter corresponding to this basal pressure was determined with a micrometric scale placed in the image plane of the microscope. A strain-gauge isotonic microdynamometer (Basile mod. MDI 4) with a load of 1 g/5 mm^2 was then set on the artery. The vessel stretching corresponding to each increase of intraluminal pressure until a maximum of 500 mm Hg was displayed on a tektronix oscilloscope and recorded on a polygraph (Elema Schonander mod. Mingograph 34). A calibration was made between voltage values and effective increases of the vessel diameter, expressed in mm. In a second group of experiments the right carotid artery was catheterized and connected to a Hewlett-Packard pressure transducer. The strain gauge was set on the other artery; the same vessel was placed on a stiff support in order not to contaminate the strain recording by respiratory movements. Blood pressure and pulse volume curve were then registered. One of two cervical vagi was isolated and cut; the distal end was electrically stimulated to achieve a strong bradycardia and an increase of pulse pressure. In both experiments CO_2 laser was used at 40 watts for 2-3 seconds with a spot size five times larger than the vessel diameter; Argon laser was used at 5 watts for 10 seconds with a spot size three times larger than the vessel diameter; Nd:YAG laser was used at 60 watts for 3 seconds with a spot size three times larger than the vessel diameter.

RESULTS

According to Gorisch[2,3] we have observed after laser irradiation a vessel constriction of about 20% without important reduction of blood flow. Macroscopic data were unchanged after 30 and 60 days in all cases treated with CO_2 and Argon laser. All vessels irradiated with Nd:YAG laser showed a complete obliteration by intraluminal thrombosis. The first figure shows the change of elastic resistance of the vessel walls in the first group of experiments, both in the acute and chronic stage. The strain degree occurring for a fixed intraluminal pressure diminishes to 51 ± 15% after laser irradiation and therefore the stress opposing the strain increases correspondingly. The increase of the elastic resistance of the irradiated vessels remains the same even at very high pressure loads. Arteries do not break even at 500 mm Hg. To obtain a more precise evaluation we have extrapolated a second curve showing tension and circumference of the vessel (Fig. 2). As it is shown by the graph with the increase of the vessel strain the tension

ssively increases and each tension value, corresponding to a fixed
n is greater after laser irradiation. The third graph (Figure 3) shows
lastic behavior of the carotid artery at different blood pressure
ond group of experiments). Evaluating a same pulse pressure the strain
ee diminishes to 65 $\pm$ 19% after laser irradiation.

LUSIONS

The exposed data show that the Argon laser and the CO_2 laser produce a
inkage of the collagen fibers and an increase in the elastic resistance
the vessel walls preserving the patency of the lumen. The Nd:YAG laser
oduces a shrinkage of the vessel and marked endothelial lesions which
acilitate the erythrocyte aggregation to the walls and the subsequent
thrombus formation. These peculiar effects seem to offer two different
possibilities for a selective vascular surgery.

268

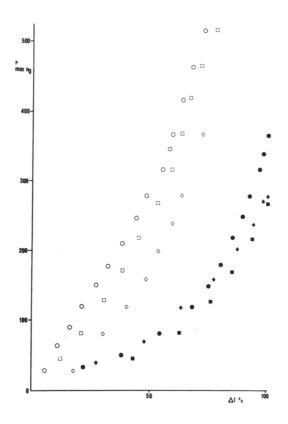

Fig.1 Effects of the laser irradiation on the vessel walls.On the
right curve before laser,on the left curve after laser.

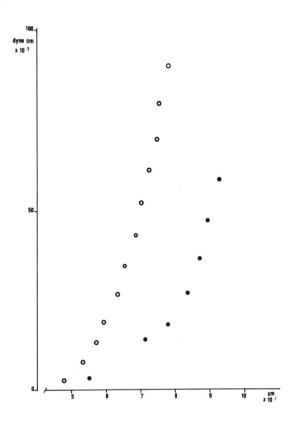

Fig.2 Effects of the laser on the vessel walls.On the right curve
before laser,on the left curve after laser.

270

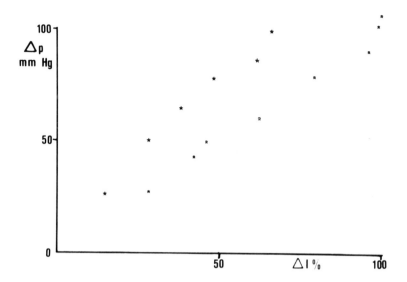

Fig.3 Effects of the laser on the vessel walls.On the right curve before laser,on the left curve after laser.

REFERENCES

1. Gorisch,W.,Boergen,K.P.,McCord,R.C.,Weinberg,W.,Hillenkamp,F. (1978) Temperature Measurements of Isolated Mesenteric Blood Vessels of the Rabbit during Laser Irradiation. Kaplan,I.ed., Jerusalem, Lasers surgery,II,pp202-207.
2. Gorisch,W.,Boergen,K.P.(1979) Thermal Shrinkage of Collagen Fibres During Vessel Occlusion in Laser Surgery. Kaplan,I.,ed., Jerusalem, Lasers surgery,III part two,pp 123-127.
3. Fasano,V.A.,Urciuoli,R.,Ponzio,R.M.(1982) Photocoagulation of Cerebral Arterio-venous Malformations and Arterial Aneurysms with the Neodymium:Yttrium-Aluminum-Garnet or Argon laser. Preliminary results in twelve Patients. Neurosurg.,11,754-760.

CHAPTER 29

PULSED Nd:YAG LASER: STUDY WITH AN INFRARED CAMERA

Principal Author:

S. Mordon
Centre de Technologie Biomedicale
INSERM S.C N°4
Lille, France

PULSED Nd. YAG LASER : STUDY WITH AN INFRARED CAMERA.

S. MORDON*, J.M. BRUNETAUD°, L. MOSQUET°, J.R. CHARLIER*, F. CARPENTIER+
J. BOUREZ°, J. MIGNE**

* Centre de Technologie Biomédicale INSERM S.C.N°4, Lille, France.
° Centre Multidisciplinaire de Traitement par laser, C.H.U., Lille, France.
+ Laboratoire d'Anatomie et de Cytologie Pathologique C. (Pr. GOSSELIN),
  Lille, France.
** Société QUANTEL, Orsay, France.

ABSTRACT

The pulsed Nd-YAG laser presents a great interest for the hemostasis of fragile tissue. The laser emission parameters should be carefully chosen in order to avoid the volatilization and hollowing at the surface and excess in necrosis in depth. Experimentations were carried out on rat liver in vivo for relating the laser parameters to the thermal effects. The control of surface temperature is achieved by an infrared camera, and the depth extension of necrosis is measured by histology.

Pulsed laser provides a better control of tissues diffusivity and surface temperature.

HEMOSTASIS AND LASER

Lasers are becoming important tools in human surgery and surgical endoscopy, finding applications as light scalpels and coagulators to stop bleeding or to coagulate tumor.

Hemostasis requires the creation of a coagulation necrosis, without volatilization. Volatilization destroys the tissues architecture and is very likely to increase the flow of the hemorrhage. Hemostasis also necessitates the adaptation of the coagulated tissue volume to the type of bleeding. A superficial coagulation, i.e. with less than 1 mm depth, is sufficient to stop capillary hemorrhage. Depth should reach 3 mm for an arteriole 2 mm diameter (3,4). For the bleeding of fragile tissues such as liver, kidney, spleen, the diameter of the exposed area should be as large as possible.

These three different coagulation effects, i.e. superficial, deep and extended, are needed in routine clinical work.

A study conducted in 1981 on dogs demonstrated that the effects of high power pulsed Nd-YAG laser were likely to satisfy the 3 types of actions described (1).

On the stomach ulcer, superficial and deep effects were obtained by choosing suitable laser emission parameter.

On fragile tissues, with a spot 1 and 2 cm in diameter, excellent and rapid hemostasis was achieved.

Preliminary experimental work provided the qualitative validation of our hypothesis, i.e. that one laser could induce the three required coagulation effects.

Quantification is necessary in order to determine the best emission parameters for each hemostasis and to avoid the main disavantage of this Nd-YAG laser, i.e. the energy overdosage. Energy overdosage can induce tissue volatilization followed by a hollowing at the surface or depth extension of necrosis with secondary infection and abcess.

The goals of this new experimental work are the control of surface temperature which must be kept under 100°C in order to avoid volatilization, and the control of necrosis depth.

MATERIALS AND METHODS -

1- Laser.
        A high power pulsed Nd-YAG laser developed by QUANTEL (Orsay, France) is used in our experiments. The laser beam is transmitted in a 400 Microns quartz fiber (Fibres Optiques Industries, Pithiviers, France). This quartz fiber allows for a transmission rate of 80 percent with a length of 4 meters. The divergent angle of the laser at the tip is about 8 degrees.
        The laser provides independent control of energy, pulse duration, delay between pulses, pulse rate. Average power can be adjusted between 10 and 150 Watts. Peak power varies from 100 to 500 Watts. Duration and delay can vary up from a few milliseconds to continuous.

2- Temperature measurement.
        The measurement system includes an infrared camera (Thermovision 720, AGA, Sweden) with a telemetric focusing system. The infrared thermography eliminates the contact with the tissue, is insensitive to the laser beam and provides good spatial and temporal resolutions (10,16).
        In order to realize a quantitative analysis of the thermal data, the frames are recorded via a modified video-recorder, digitalized and processed by a microcomputer (14).
        Thermal data can be visualized as temperature profile (spatial distribution of the thermal energy at a given time) and temperature evolution at a given position in the frame during 8 seconds.

3- Methods.
        Liver of Wistar male rats were used for the experiments, providing an homogeneous medium. A 2 mm in diameter laser beam with uniform energy distribution was used. One day after laser irradiation, the rats were sacrified and submitted to histological examination, including necrosis depth measurement and a qualitative analysis of necrosis structure.

RESULTS -

        Experiments performed on 30 rats provided 140 laser irradiation sequences. Theses laser irradiation sequences were analyzed according to 3 criteria :
                1- Reproductivity and reliability ;
                2- Quantitative analysis of single laser shots ;
                3- Quantitative analysis of multiple laser shots ;

1- Reproductivity and reliability.
        Reproductivity of the thermal data obtained by the infrared measures and the computer data acquisition were verified. Identical surface temperatures were found with identical laser irradiation parameters.
        For each experiment, temperature curves obtained were well correlated to corresponding histological data.

2- Single laser shots.
        Of the140 laser irradiation sequences analyzed, 83 corresponded to a single laser shots. Surface temperature and necrosis were studied with energy density ranging from 150 to 300 J/cm^2, peak power from 100 to 180 Watts and irradiation duration from 30 to 200 milliseconds. In this case, temperature increased linearly with the energy density, independently of laser parameters such as peak power and laser irradiation duration (Fig. 1).
        At temperatures below 100°C, the histological cuts showed that necrosis volume increases linearly with the energy density. Depth necrosis is related to laser pulse duration and to peak power density.

3- Multiple laser shots.

The goals of this study were to evaluate the effects of high power Nd.YAG laser rapid pulse sequences, to determine the influence of the delay between pulses on the temporal surface temperature gradient and the necrosis 2,3 or 4 laser shots.

We established that the temporal surface temperature gradient was proportional to the ratio duration over delay between pulses.

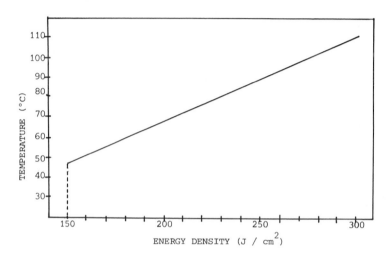

Figure 1 : Surface temperature as a function of energy density Nd. YAG power : 100-180W, irradiation time 30-200 ms, beam diamter : 2 mm.

DISCUSSION -

1- Single shots.

The results concerning the relationship between surface temperature and energy density are in agreement with those obtained by other investigation who are using longer pulse durations (over 1 second).

Mc CORD (13) has obtained 59°C for an energy density of 185/cm^2 ; CASTRO (2), 58°C for 170 J/cm^2 ; HOFFSTETTER (9), 60°C for 180 J/cm^2 and IWASAKI (13), 100°C for 300 J/cm^2.

The results concerning the relationship between energy density and volume necrosis, and between power density and necrosis depth are in agreement with ROTHENBERGER (17). He demonstrated that with constant power and increasing time, the width of necrosis increases and its depth remains constant.

The results are also in agreement with HALLDORSSON and LANGERHOLC's results (5,6,7,12). They showed that scattering increased with energy density and peak power defined the depth of volume scattering.

Volume scattering is mainly characterized by the reduction of the beam penetration, the redistribution of energy at the surface and the volume broadening.

2- Multiple shots.

The influence of the delay between pulses on the temporal gradient was described by Mc. CORD and PENSEL (15) as directly related to surface

temperature. It allows for a control of volatilization of necrosis extension volume. The heat distribution is determined by the heat conduction law
(8).

$$q(r,t) = Jt/JT - A \quad J^2/J^2T$$

$q(r,t)$: temperature distribution at any position and time ;
t : time, T : temperature, r : position, A : thermal diffusivity.

In this equation, the thermal diffusiveness characterizes the tissues
and is related to the inter-pulse delay.

$$A = f(t_1/t_1 + t_2)$$

t_1 : pulse duration, t_2 : delay between pulses.

Tissues are coagulated when heated at a temperature for a specific
time interval. The damage degree is defined to be less or equal to 1, if
tissue damage is reversible, and greater to 1 if it is irreversibly
damaged. In order to achieve a perfect coagulation, the temperature has to
be kept constant during a given time. This is very difficult to achieve
with CW lasers. However, the adaptation of t_1 and t_2 allows to reach a
steady state during the coagulation.

CONCLUSION -

The described system which allows the acquisition and data proces-
sing of thermal data, is reliable . Thermal interaction between laser light
and tissue is the main mechanism in medical applications of lasers and a
quantitative determination of thermal effects provides an important contribution to the optimization of emitting parameters.
The present study has demonstrated that previous results obtained
with low power and long irradiation time were still valid under higher
power levels and shorter time durations. Such a high power pulsed Nd. YAG
laser presents two advantages over the conventional CW lasers. The spot
diameter can be very large, which is important for fragile tissues. The
controlability of pulse duration and pulse rate allows to maintain a steady
surface temperature during treatment and provides an adequate control of
the coagulation process.

REFERENCES -

1. BRUNETAUD J.M., MIGNE J., BETTOUART M., BISERTE J., BOUREZ J., CHARLIER
   J., LEROUX J., VANDENBUSCHE P.
   Hémostase et laser Yag-Neodyme impulsionnel. OPTO 81, 1981.
2. CASTRO D., STUART A., BENVENUTI D., DWYER R., LEVASOY M.A. A new method
   of densitometry : a study of comparative laser induced tissue damage.
   Proc. 4th Int. Congress of Laser Surgery, Tokyo, 1981.
3. EICHLER J., KNOF J., LENZ H. Measurements on the depth of penetration
   of light (0,35-1,0ym) in tissue. Rad.& Environm.Biophys., 1977, 239-242.
4. EICHLER J. KNOF J., LENZ J., SALK J., SCHAFER G. Temperature distribution in tissue during laser irradiation. Rad.& Environm.,1978,15,277-287.
5. HALLDORSSON Th., LANGERHOLC J. Thermodynamic analysis of laser irradiation of biological tissue. Applied Optics, 1978, 17, 24, 3948-3958.
6. HALLDORSSON Th., LANGERHOLC J., KROY W., SENATORI L. Interaction of
   laser light with biological tissue. Proc.3rd Int.Congress of Laser
   surgery, Graz, 1979.
7. HALLDORSSON Th., ROTHER W., LANGERHOLC J., FRANK F. Theoretical and
   experimental investigations prove Nd. YAG laser treatment to be safe.
   Lasers In Surgery and Medicine, 1981, 1, 253-262.

8. HAVERKAMPF K., MEYER H., LUDOLPH M., ELBERT B. Basic investigations about different types of lasers in surgery. Proc. 3rd Int Congress of Laser Sugery, Graz, 1979.
9. HOSTETTER A. The Nd. YAG laser in urology. The Journal of Japan Society for laser Medicine, Vol. 1, N°1.
10. HSIEH C.K., ELINGTON W.A. A quantitative determination of surface temperatures using an infrared camera. SPIE, 1977, 124, 228-235.
11. IWASAKI M., KONISHI T., MURATA N., MARUYAMA Y., WADA T. Effect of argon and YAG lasers on canine esophagus. Proc.3rd. Int.Congress of Laser Surgery, Graz, 1979.
12. LANGERHOLC J. Moving phase transitions in laser irradiated biological tissue. Applied Optics, 1979, 18, 13, 2286-2293.
13. MC.CORD R.C., WEINBERG W., GORISH W., LEMETA F., SCHONBERGER J.L., Thermal effects in laser irradiated biological tissues. Proc. 3rd. Int Congress of Laser, Graz, 1979.
14. MORDON S., CHARLIER J.R., BRUNETAUD J.M., MOSCHETTO Y. Acquisition et traitement d'images obtenues en thermographie infrarouge pour l'étude des effects thermiques des lasers sur les tissus vivants. Innov. Tech. Biol. Med., 1981, 4,2, 183-193.
15. PENSEL J. HOFSTETTER A., KEIDITSCH E., ROTHENBERGER K., STAEHLER G., FRANK F., GORISH W. Temperature profile in space and time on the bladder wall serosa during intravesical laser irradiation. Proc. 3rd. Int Gongress of Laser, Graz, 1979.
16. REED R.D., MIKESELL G.W. Radiometer monitoring of exposure-site temperature during laser irradiation. Phys. Med. Biol., 1981, 26, 1, 175-180.
17. ROTHENBERGER K., PENSEL J. HOFSTETTER A., FRANK F., KEIDITSH E., STEN J. Dosimetry of the Neodynium-Yag Laser in endovesical application. Proc. Int. Congress of laser surgery, Tokyo, 1981.

282